# Choices and Consequences

## BY TODD CRANDELL

### CO-AUTHORED BY LAUREN KANNE

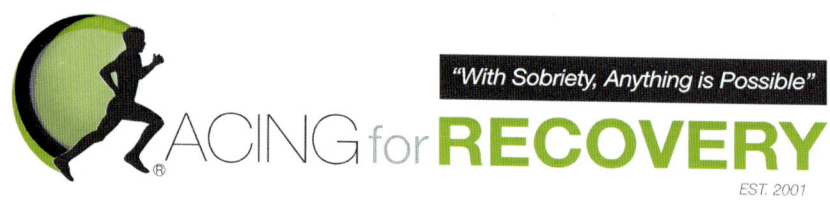

"With Sobriety, Anything is Possible"

ACING for **RECOVERY**

EST. 2001

© 2019 Todd Crandell

Published by Racing for Recovery
6202 Trust Drive, Holland, Ohio 43528
www.racingforrecovery.org
419.824.8462

Design by Marlene Schmitt
www.TheImageGroup.net

ISBN: 978-1-7334937-0-3

# CONTENTS

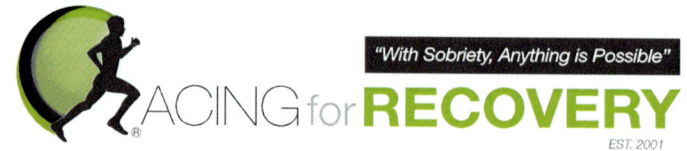
"With Sobriety, Anything is Possible"

ACING for RECOVERY

EST. 2001

# ACKNOWLEDGMENTS

With grace and gratitude I would like to thank the following people for making this book possible. God, my family, friends and the awesome "staff" at Racing for Recovery for all you do to make my life what it is.

To my co-author Lauren Kanne, thank you for believing in my story and the Racing for Recovery mission. It has been a pleasure working with you and I appreciate your kindness, intelligence and passion for this book.

To Marlene Schmitt from The Image Group, thank you for your creativity and expertise in making the look of this book possible. You are an extremely talented individual.

Last but not least, I thank YOU the reader. Because you are reading this, not only do I wish you are helped in some capacity but that you share this with another individual who can do the same.

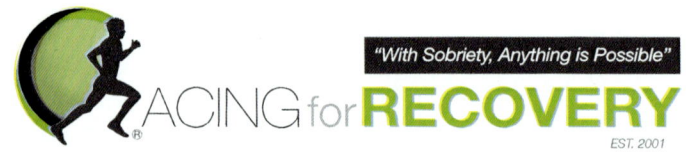

## DEDICATION

This book is dedicated to the youth, the individual in recovery, families, educators, clergy, first responders, healthcare professionals, coaches, or anyone who faces difficult emotional decisions daily.

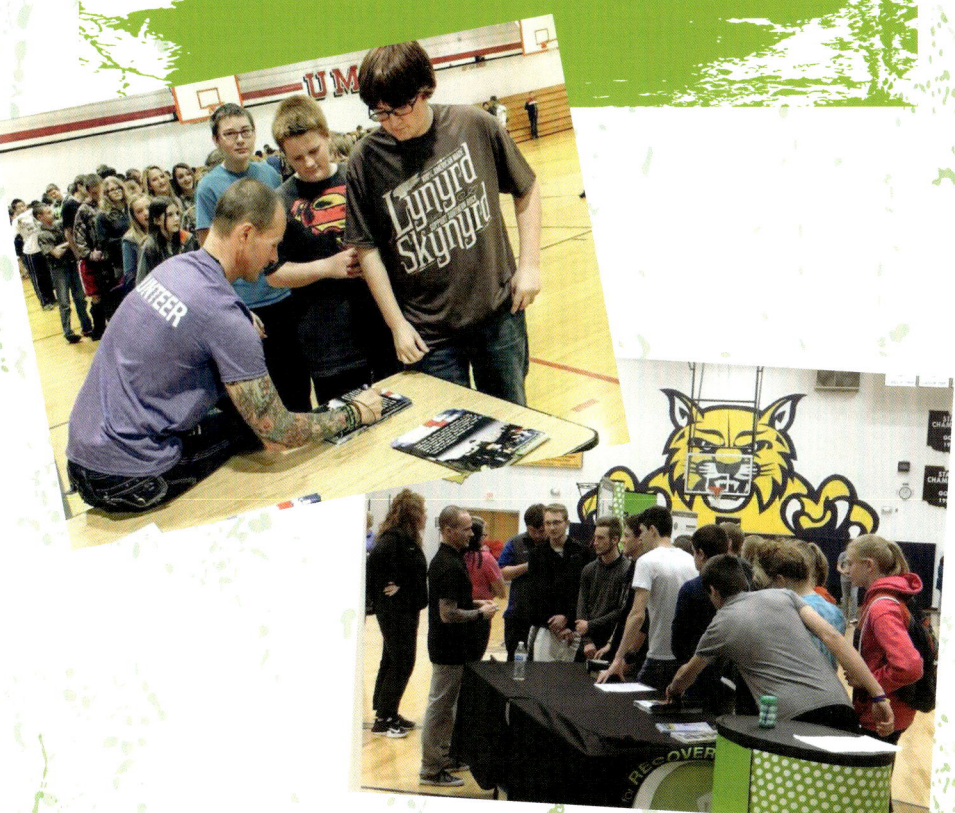

## STEVIN GROTH
## GROTH & ASSOCIATES, PARTNER, ATTORNEY

I have known and worked with Todd Crandell and Racing for Recovery for many years. As a former prosecutor and long-time criminal defense attorney here in Northwest Ohio, I have seen the dramatic shift from punishment via incarceration to effective treatment methods in our justice system. This is true on a state and local level. In many ways, the legal system is just now catching up to what Racing for Recovery has been focused on from its very start—treating the root cause of addiction, rather than merely treating the addiction itself.

This system-wide change in focusing on the underlying cause of addiction has only taken place in recent years. As opiate addiction reached crisis levels, the legal system desperately looked for new ways to change the cycle of incarceration and death. Racing for Recovery was ahead of the curve in understanding that addiction is rooted in deeper personal issues. The Racing for Recovery Model has become a framework for other agencies and courts to utilize.

However, there is a natural tension among the three parts of the system involved with an individual's life: the State, the defense attorneys, and the treatment providers. The State (prosecution and judges), on some level, need to punish people for illegal behavior. The defense attorney is tasked with minimizing punishment. Treatment providers like Racing for Recovery want to engage the person with the necessary services to find sobriety and stability. Each entity operating for different aims, despite really wanting the same outcome.

Fortunately, both the State and defense attorneys have come to see that the old methods weren't always effective. Tragic results of cyclical drug and alcohol abuse have led deaths to spike in alarming numbers. The Racing for Recovery model, developed by Todd Crandell, took the core idea of addressing the underlying issues, and made it part of the vernacular of both the State and the Defense.

No longer merely wanting to punish, nor wanting to skirt the issues, both sides have often joined together in a united approach to truly solve these pressing issues. Of course, both sides fulfill their professional roles in these matters. Drug dealers and those responsible for more serious behavior are

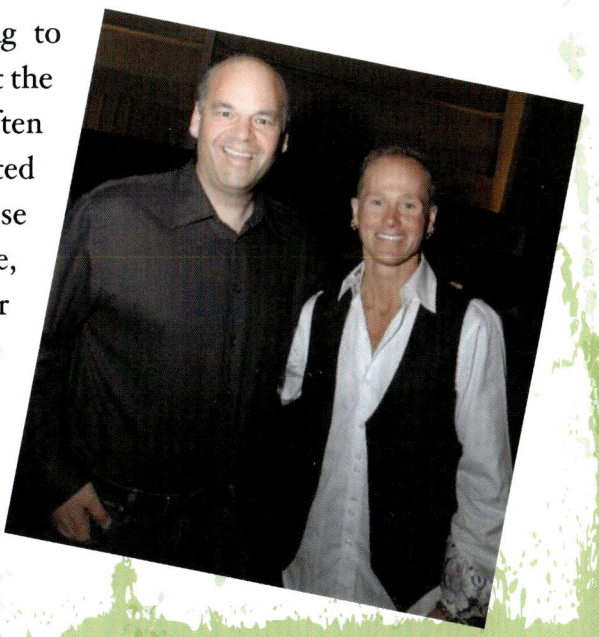

subject to punishment, and defense attorneys serve to safeguard constitutional rights and work for their clients to be certain the charges are merited. But where warranted, the clear effort is to save lives—not waste them—through treatment and counseling of the whole person in the Racing for Recovery model.

Stevin Groth
Attorney at Law
Groth & Associates
July, 2019

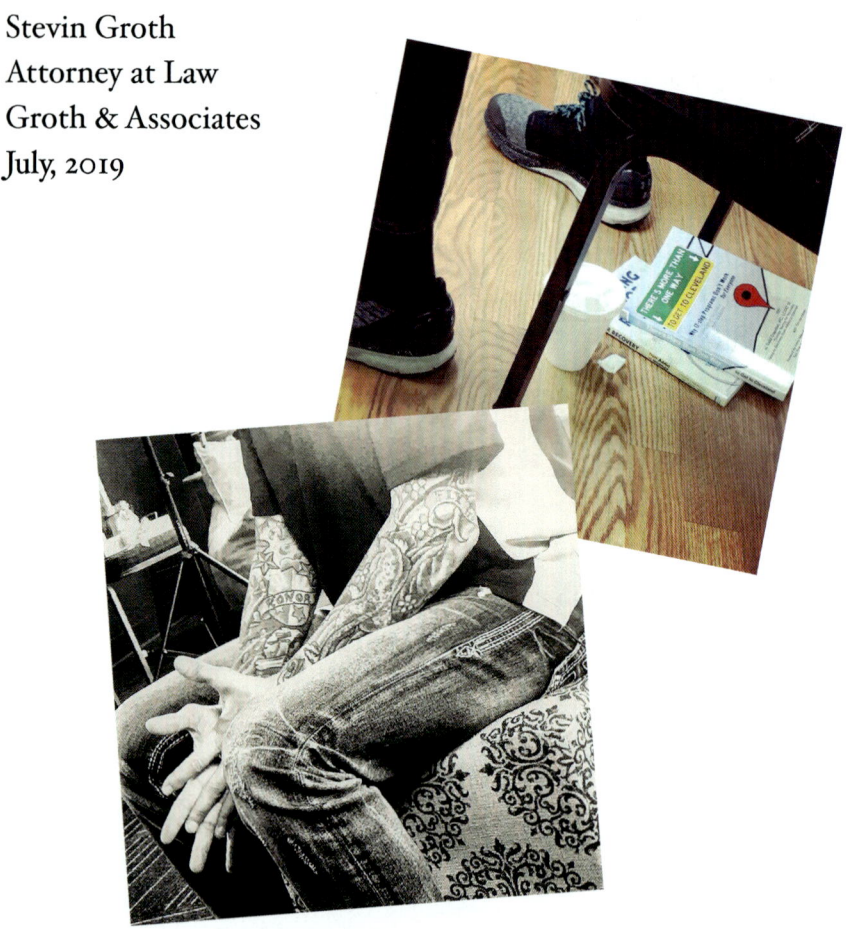

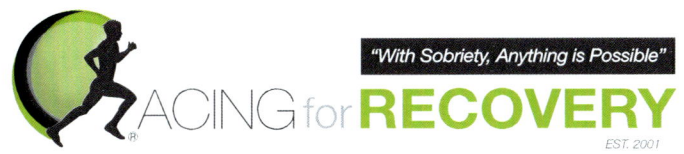

"With Sobriety, Anything is Possible"

RACING for RECOVERY

EST. 2001

# WHY ARE YOU HERE AND HOW CAN WE HELP?

Hey, you're awesome!

Yeah, I'm talking to you. Don't look so surprised—it can't be the first time you've heard that today! Have you passed by a mirror yet? I can't believe you can see your reflection without giving yourself a shout-out.

No, I'm not crazy or mistaken. You're fantastic!

Okay, you might not feel awesome right now. Actually, you seem worried. Maybe you haven't been making the choices you deserve, or maybe it's someone you love. You definitely have a lot of questions. Something is making you feel sick, sad, and afraid, and you're looking for answers.

You've come to the right place.

I wake up every morning to new emails, phone calls, Facebook messages, and drop-in visits from people facing exactly what you're going through right now. I spend all day helping them make the best choices of their lives.

From the moment we open the doors each day to the time we head home, our three phone lines ring non-stop. Rachel and Dan are usually up front, juggling all the incoming calls and people walking in. They know what it's like to feel the way you do. Everyone who works here started off looking for these answers.

We greet everyone with the same two questions: why are you here and how can we help?

## WAIT—WHO ARE YOU TO TELL ME ANYTHING?

That's a fair question—I guess I should introduce myself!

I'm Todd Crandell. I'm a licensed professional clinical counselor with supervision designation (LPCC-S) and a licensed independent chemical dependency counselor clinical supervisor (LICDC-CS). That means I earned a master's degree studying why people behave the way they do, especially in regards to drugs and alcohol. Then, I spent a lot of time helping people with their addictions in a clinical setting—so much time that now, I'm even allowed to train and supervise other people who want to help. Then, I took some (really hard) tests to prove I knew my stuff.

Sharing the Racing for Recovery mission with students in Kentucky

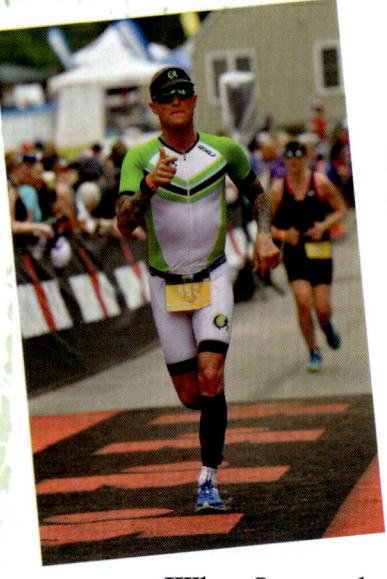

I'm also an extreme athlete. I ran my first IRONMAN triathlon on November 6, 1999, to prove to myself that with sobriety, anything is possible. As of summer 2019, I've traveled all over the world to finish two ULTRAMAN races, thirty IRONMAN races, and forty-seven IRONMAN 70.3 triathlons.

When I started running, the press quickly picked up on my story. I was amazed by how many people found hope in my message, and I knew I needed to do more. So, in 2001, I founded Racing for Recovery, a group that empowers people to live healthy, happy, sober, and balanced lives. It started with weekly support meetings, and it's grown and evolved to help thousands of people and their families. We're a huge community now with our own facilities, offering counseling, housing, classes, and programs seven days a week. We offer a lot of resources in person and online, including webinars,

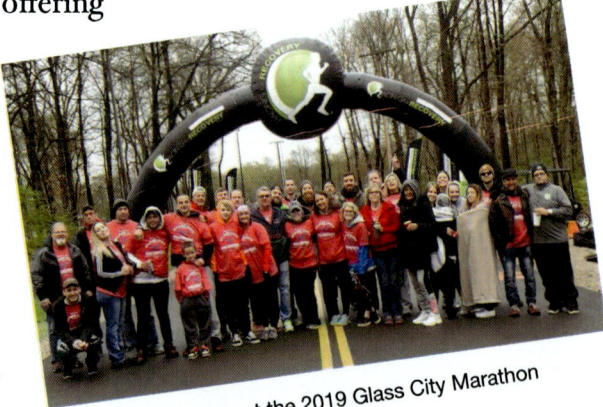

Volunteering at the 2019 Glass City Marathon

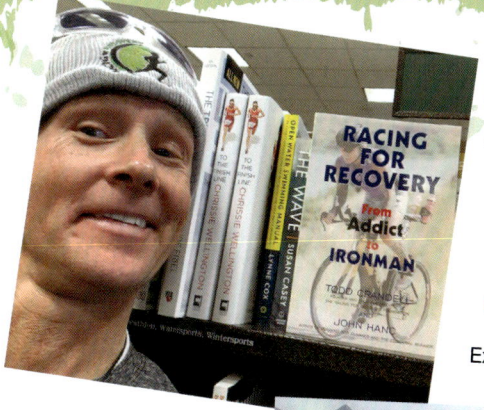

IRONMAN Chattanooga 70.3 with Racing for Recovery Executive Director, Todd Bieber, and two success stories

videos, and meetings. We just finished filming our third documentary, and this is the third book I've written.

I'm surrounded by incredible people each and every day. I work side-by-side with the most inspirational, dedicated team I can imagine. My friends and I go on huge adventures across the globe with rock stars. I go home to my wonderful wife, Melissa, four awesome kids, and a whole menagerie of pets (including Milo, the pig).

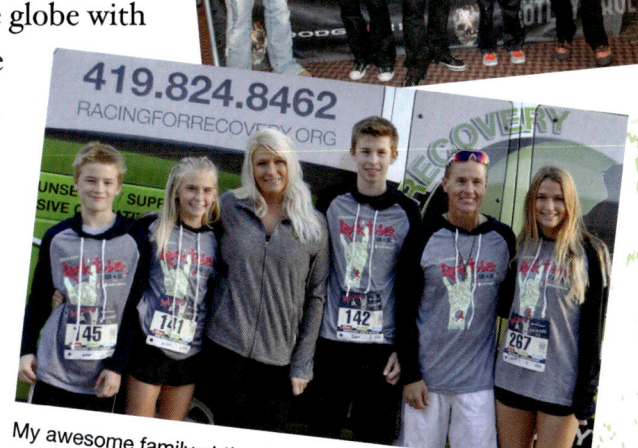

My awesome family at the 2017 Racing for Recovery 5K event

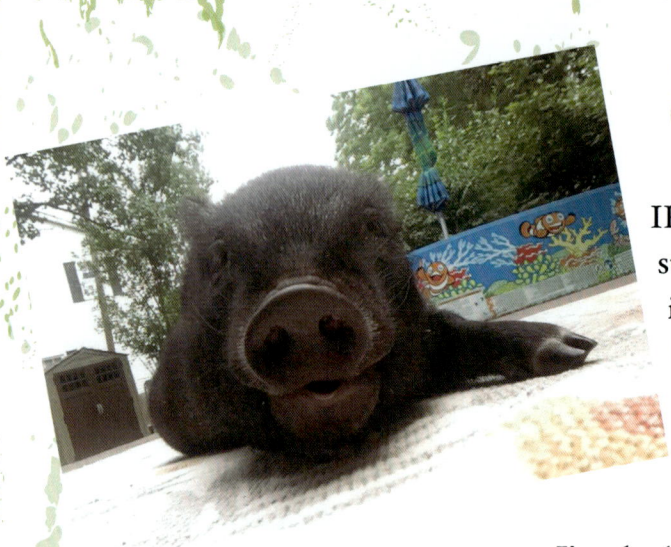

IRONMAN? Rock stars? Pig?!?! Now it sounds like I'm bragging. Some guys are just born lucky, right?

Maybe, but that's not me. I'm the "luckiest" guy in the world now. Before that, I made all sorts of bad **CHOICES** and faced terrible **CONSEQUENCES.**

I know what it's like to be so lost, you're sure you'll never find your way out. I know what it's like to feel worthless. I know what it's like to get kicked out of school, to destroy all your relationships, to flush your future down the drain. I know what it's like to want to die. For thirteen years, I caved in to pain and let drugs run my life into the ground.

## FOUR BIG CHOICES

Many people don't kick addiction to the curb with conventional treatment methods. The percentage of people who begin using again after treatment hovers somewhere around 80%.

On paper, I look like one of the success stories. I went through conventional treatment, and I have been drug-free now for twenty-six years (over a quarter of a century!). I've even devoted my life to addiction and sobriety.

I wouldn't be here if I'd continued to make the decisions I was making towards drugs, alcohol, and life in general. The truth is, though, that I didn't find the key to my sobriety in those conventional treatments either. If I had just followed the programs, I wouldn't have the life I have today. If that type of thinking had "stuck," I would still be where I was in 1993— hopefully sober, but still in a lot of pain.

Have you ever heard, "The harder I worked, the luckier I got"? Well, in my experience, that just doesn't hold totally true. Your hard work has to be aimed in the right direction. I don't think many people understand motivation, determination, focus, and drive as well as people with addictions. I used to work really hard trying to cover my pain with drugs and alcohol; once I chose sobriety, I worked hard towards being a pharmaceutical rep; once I realized my life's mission, I worked really hard to get "my own way."

None of those choices made me "lucky."

I got "lucky" and built the incredible life I have today once I started making the right choices across four different categories—

## CHOOSING SOBRIETY, CHOOSING TO HEAL, CHOOSING LOVE, AND CHOOSING TO PURSUE MY PASSION.

This book has a lot of different components, but when we boil it down, it's about decisions we all have to make in those four categories. I'll share some real stories about making the wrong choice and facing the consequences and some science and insight about why so many of us are attracted to these bad decisions.

I'm not here to scare you into doing the right thing. I'm also going to show you how the whole world opens up to you when you make the right choices. At this point, I've got it down to a foolproof formula: if you do A, you will get B. The path to a holistic, happy, well-balanced lifestyle is pretty simple, but you don't stumble across it by accident. It takes a lot of work, but the results are incredible! When you make the right choices, life is better (and never, ever boring).

My accomplishments in life and with Racing for Recovery might look enormous. No joke—that's because they are. But they aren't unattainable. You can accomplish things this cool and better, and you don't even have to search for the secrets for a quarter of a century. It's all laid out in this book for you. I'm giving you a detailed plan of how to do it. I've taken this awesome thing and broken it down into the choices that you have to make along the way to get here. It's all bite-size and attainable.

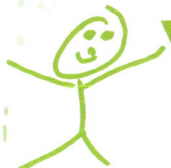

No way!

I promote Racing for Recovery through the media a lot, but at this point, most people learn about us through other people we've helped. Every day, we hear some variation of, "Hey, my cousin/sibling/friend told me you're different and awesome and changed his/her life, and I really need that…"

Yes, I started the program and I still play a big role in it, but it is so much bigger than me and my story now. Nothing makes me prouder and happier than the many other people building off of these principles to create their own incredible lives and accomplish amazing things. All the clients don't just work with me anymore—they seek out the counselors with the gifts and stories they relate to. I love it when somebody comes in with no idea who I am. (It's actually a running joke around here that I'm the janitor.)

To bring that energy into this book and give you more perspectives on what these choices look like in other people's lives, I've asked several members of the Racing for Recovery team to contribute their own stories in their own words.

We are a team of real, awesome people who have experienced many different types of trauma. The one thing we all have in common is that we were once so positive we weren't awesome that we tried to hide from ourselves and from the world with alcohol and drugs. It didn't work for us then (and it won't work for you now). We've made bad choices and faced the consequences of them. We know how to turn lives around, because we did it ourselves. We've done everything that seemed impossible when we were in the grips of trauma and addiction. And we're here to show you how.

## WHOA, WHY DO YOU THINK DRUGS ARE A PROBLEM IN MY LIFE?!

Well, statistically...they are.

- *Percent of persons aged 12 years and over with any illicit drug use in the past month: 10.6% (2016)*

- *In 2015, 26.9 percent of people ages 18 or older reported that they engaged in binge drinking in the past month; 7.0 percent reported that they engaged in heavy alcohol use in the past month.*

- *15.1 million adults ages 18 and older (6.2 percent of this age group) had diagnosed addiction issues. This includes 9.8 million men (8.4 percent of men in this age group) and 5.3 million women (4.2 percent of women in this age group).*

- *About 6.7 percent of adults who had diagnosed*

*addiction issues in the past year received treatment. This includes 7.4 percent of males and 5.4 percent of females in this age group.*

*• An estimated 623,000 adolescents ages 12–17 (2.5 percent of this age group) had diagnosable addiction issues. This number includes 298,000 males (2.3 percent of males in this age group) and 325,000 females (2.7 percent of females in this age group).*

*• About 5.2 percent of youth who had diagnosable addiction issues in the past year received treatment. This includes 5.1 percent of males and 5.3 percent of females with AUD in this age group.*

If you're facing problems with addiction or you're at risk, you're certainly not alone. This book is for you. I'm going to walk you through the choices you need to get and stay balanced, healthy, and sober.

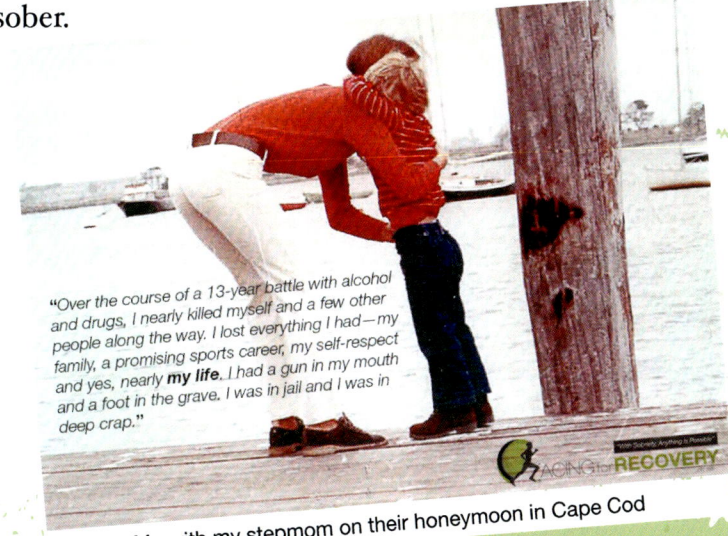

"Over the course of a 13-year battle with alcohol and drugs, I nearly killed myself and a few other people along the way. I lost everything I had—my family, a promising sports career, my self-respect and yes, nearly **my life**. I had a gun in my mouth and a foot in the grave. I was in jail and I was in deep crap."

Me with my stepmom on their honeymoon in Cape Cod

If you love someone who has problems with addiction, this book is for you. I'm going to explain things about addiction and sobriety that really confuse, scare, and anger people who have never had problems with addiction and show you how you can help.

If you've never touched drugs and never will and you never even meet someone with an addiction, that's awesome—but this book is also for you. Believe it or not, all sorts of people without any drug problems love coming to Racing for Recovery. The stories and tips I'm going to share are motivating, healthy, and will help to make your life better, no matter what you face.

Drugs and alcohol are a huge problem, and we're going to talk a lot about them, but they're also symptoms of some bigger issues that affect everyone. You're going to face hard decisions in your life, and no one makes the right ones on the first try every single time. At some point, we all feel bad about ourselves, and we all try to cover over problems in our lives rather than dealing with them. People and circumstances influence you, but your life is 100% your responsibility. A lot of people never really learn that, but "lucky" people do (usually the hard way), and use it to build great lives—the type you want to live. I'll help you build a skill set that scales to fit every decision.

This is the book I wanted when I was young and confused and in so much pain. This is the book I wish I could have handed to my parents, friends, teachers, and doctors, to help explain what was going on inside my head and why it was coming out in my behaviors and actions.

No matter who you are or what you're facing, being awesome is a full-time job. I'm going to show you how to be the best you—physically, emotionally, intellectually, and socially.

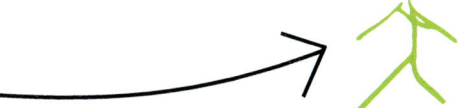

## WHO IS THIS GUY?

Oh, me. And you. Everybody, really. The DUDE represents us as individuals in the journey of self betterment and the different emotions we think, feel and express. I have no artistic ability (as illustrated by the DUDE), but I use the whiteboard a lot in the educational groups I am fortunate to conduct. The DUDE has become a thing over the past few years, sort of an unofficial mascot that Racing for Recovery people relate to and expect to see during our sessions.

The DUDE makes frequent appearances in this book to keep us grounded in the moment. We're going to be dealing with some pretty serious stuff (life is always full of serious stuff), but no matter what you're facing at the moment, there's joy in there too (life is always full of joy, even in the most serious stuff).

The DUDE will walk us through it all so we've always got someone to high-five, even when things get serious.

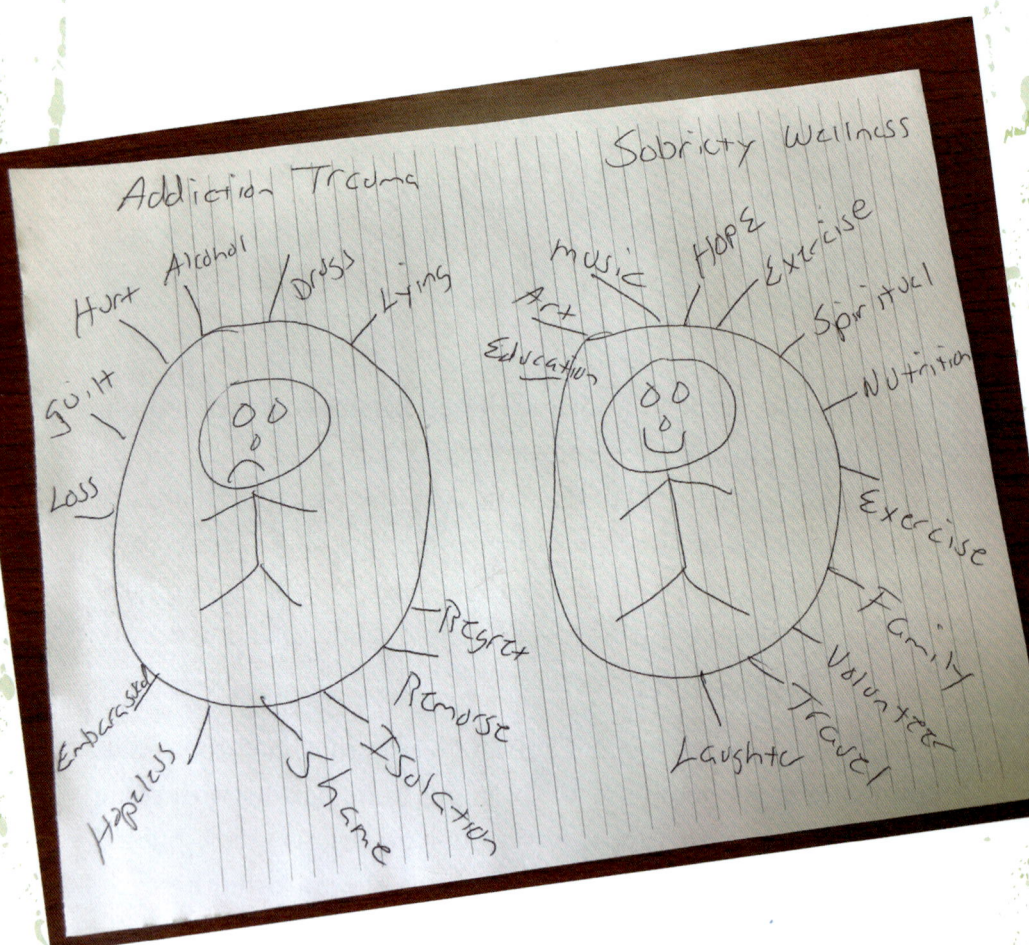

## HOW DO I USE THIS BOOK?

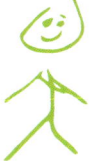

A new client showed up at our intensive outpatient group the other day, so, of course, she got the two-question treatment:

### "HI! WHY ARE YOU HERE AND HOW CAN WE HELP?"

She looked really confused for a second, which confused me. Did I get my wires crossed?

"Wow! No one has ever asked me that question," she finally responded.

A smile flickered across her face, and a glimmer of hope in her eyes struck me right in the heart. I can never forget walking into rooms like this for the first time, feeling broken, worthless, beat up, and desperate to be seen.

A lot of people have big ideas about how to help with addiction—and the people who are struggling often get buried under those ideas. Why are you here and how can we help are two short questions that say as much as they ask:

**I AM INTERESTED IN LISTENING TO YOU. I VALUE YOUR THOUGHTS ON YOUR OWN ISSUES, AND I RESPECT YOU AND YOUR DIGNITY. YOU'RE THE BOSS.** I've been learning new things about recovery every day for many years, but people are way more than the sum of their addictions. I always recognize that you are the world's leading expert on you.

If you walked into Racing for Recovery for the first time, you'd tell us about yourself, what you're facing, and what you want help with. Then, we would set you up with an individualized treatment plan. Everyone needs different things at different times—some people come in just needing help with one particular thing, while other people want to take part in a much more extensive program.

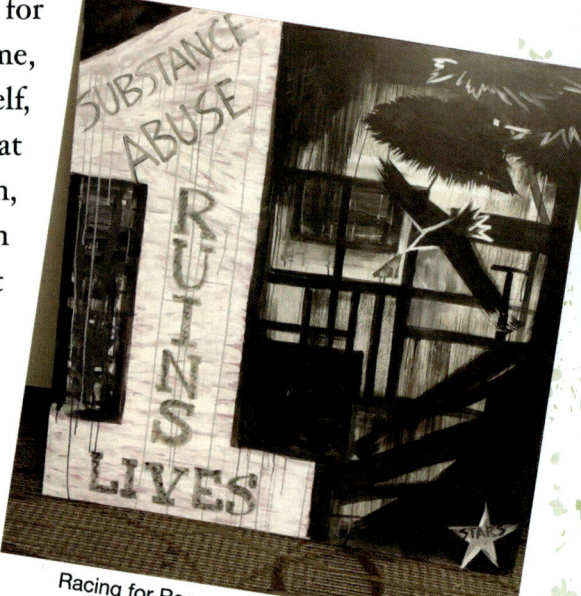

Racing for Recovery Lifestyle Number One

From the moment someone asks for help, we start figuring out the ways—medically, physically, emotionally, and psychologically—to get them. (Our program is holistic, which means we're committed to helping each person access the services they need to get their act together, even if we don't provide them in-house. We are always looking for ways to say 'yes.') Of course, I highly recommend that everyone take advantage of everything we offer, because it will change their lives and the way they think. But I'm not trying to force or trap anyone, and I can't change parts of people's lives they don't want (or are not ready) to change. Your individual plan would be modified as your needs and focus changed.

I've set up this book the same way. You can read it cover to cover and get a good sense of a whole mindset shift that can change your life and the way you understand your problems. Or, you can pinpoint the topic that is causing you acute pain (or just have questions about). You don't have to buy into everything right away—take the guidance you find in the section that you believe relates most to your life at the moment, apply it, and watch your life start to change. Once you realize how good that feels, you can always come back for more.

*You're an awesome person, and I really believe you're going to make great choices. Make one right now—turn the page and get started.*

Todd Crandell
March 2019

(Man, I knew I was right about you. AWESOME!)

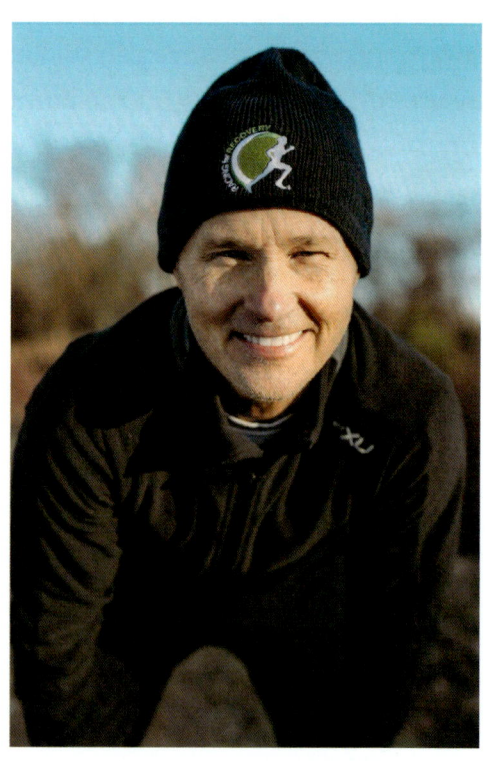

# CHOOSE SOBRIETY

Recovery is like building a house—you don't start with the roof, you start with a solid foundation. That solid foundation is getting sober.

Sobriety is the first challenge you face in any recovery program. What makes Racing for Recovery different is that it is our jumping off point, not our end goal. It's in our motto—with sobriety, anything is possible! To get to the best parts of "anything," though, we've got to get and stay sober.

In this section, we're going to talk about sobriety as a choice, take a look at some of the reasons why it is such an important choice to make, and share some stories about the consequences of not making it.

## ISN'T ADDICTION A DISEASE?

Many of us have heard that addiction is a disease so often and from so many sources that we just accept it as an undisputed fact. It's often called a disease by very kind, knowledgeable people who care greatly about people who are struggling with addictions. Believe it or not, though, addiction's "disease" status is hotly debated and highly political.

Classifying addiction as a disease became popular in the 1950s, when governmental organizations like the National Institute of Drug Abuse (NIDA) and powerful private organizations, like the American Medical Association (AMA) and Alcoholics Anonymous (AA), started promoting the Minnesota Model. The Minnesota Model, which deals exclusively with alcohol addiction, defines alcoholism as an "involuntary disability."

Although the Minnesota Model continues to form the backbone for the most popular understanding of addiction, it is one theory among many. There are thoughtful, intelligent arguments against labeling addiction a disease, and several models that seem to better fit the realities that I've experienced, both in my personal journey and as a clinician. These theories get attention within the recovery community, but they rarely get much traction in the public eye.

I believe that some of the people and organizations that heavily influence keeping this debate under a cone of silence have good intentions. Before the Minnesota Model was adopted, our society mostly believed that addictions were a moral failing of individuals who were just bad, lazy, weak, or crazy. No one who cares about people struggling with addictions wants to go back to that!

The unfortunate truth, though, is that money makes the world go 'round—and there are many people and organizations that are making a lot of money off the idea that addiction is a disease. That financial and political reality includes the fact that, with the way the insurance system is currently set up, in order for treatment to be covered, addiction (or "substance use disorder," as it is now officially named) needs to be classified as a disease.

Addiction is real, and it is dangerous. I could have easily lost my life to it many times. Addiction drove my mother to suicide when I was just three years old. I have known and mourned many who did not recover.

But, as someone who used to have serious drug and alcohol addictions and as someone who spends my days helping people choose balanced, healthy, holistic, and sober lives, I think labeling addiction as an involuntary disability/disorder/disease causes more harm than most people realize. Thinking of myself as a diseased addict, helpless and out-of-control, didn't work for me. It made me feel ashamed and worthless. When I took responsibility for myself and took control of my actions, I was able to stop drinking and using drugs and accomplish great things in life.

It's valuable for us to think about addiction outside of our understanding of disease—and certainly outside the concept of "involuntary." Blinking is involuntary. Going out, getting drugs or alcohol, and then using them is not only a choice—it is usually a series of many choices. When we hear "disease," we tend to think of something outside of our control. I would like to live in a world where we hear "addiction" and think of something preventable and fixable.

Language is important, and it shapes the way we think about ourselves and the world around us. One of the many problems with using language like "disease," "disorder," "alcoholic," or "addict" is that people start identifying with their diagnoses. When people start to see the things they are struggling with as part of their identities, they can seem permanent, not like issues that can be dealt with and choices they can make differently. At Racing for Recovery, we've created a very positive community that truly believes that with sobriety, anything is possible. One of my many proud moments recently was going around in a meeting for introductions; 137 people introduced themselves, and not one called themselves an addict or an alcoholic. We just don't make a space for that type of stigma, shame, and guilt.

**TO EFFECTIVELY FACE DOWN ADDICTION, YOU NEED ACCOUNTABILITY, RESPONSIBILITY, AND PERSEVERANCE.** With those commitments to yourself and a community that empowers you with understanding, compassion, and support, you can thrive. In my experience (and I've had a lot!), most people with addictions are treating symptoms of an underlying problem. By viewing addiction as a choice, we're able to look hard and figure out why each person who comes to us for help is making that choice. When we're able to pinpoint the underlying issue, we can treat the real problem—the reason someone started drinking or drugging in the first place.

**THINKING ABOUT ADDICTION AS A CHOICE IS EMPOWERING, BECAUSE WE CONTROL OUR CHOICES—EVEN THE MOST DIFFICULT ONES.** Imagine what a gift it would be to have the ability to cure yourself of diseases like congenital heart failure or cancer by choosing not to have them! At Racing for Recovery, we know no one is powerless in the face of addiction; we can all choose to never drink or use drugs again.

## WHY DO PEOPLE START ABUSING DRUGS AND ALCOHOL IN THE FIRST PLACE?

I started using drugs and alcohol because, on September 23, 1970, a black Pontiac Bonneville drove into a concrete abutment under a bridge, and a twenty-three-year-old woman made history as the first recorded vehicular suicide in Ohio.

I wasn't in the car; the driver was alone. I wasn't there to see it— no one was. And I certainly didn't start drinking and using drugs that night. I was only three. I've tried many times, but I can't even remember the driver, my mother, Louise Swab Crandell.

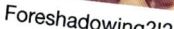

But the trauma of that event has radiated throughout my entire life. Picking up my first drink ten years later was an attempt to medicate that pain away. It didn't work, but I spent thirteen years trying, with every combination of drugs and alcohol I could get my hands on.

There are as many reasons for using drugs and alcohol as there are people who become addicted. Everyone who struggles with addiction is facing pain in their life they don't want to experience and cannot make go away.

About 90% of the people who come to Racing for Recovery seeking help for drug or alcohol addiction can trace their decisions back to some type of trauma in their childhoods. The other 10% have addictions that often began when their doctors prescribed drugs to numb them from the effects of painful medical conditions and procedures. My counselors and I

Foreshadowing?!?

call this breakdown the 90-10 Concept, and we use it to help people discover the roots of their addictions. When people can locate the place their pain originated, they can start to heal, rather than attempting to manage it with drugs and alcohol. It doesn't matter whether you're in the 90% or the 10%—if you don't go back and heal or find a healthier way to cope with the part of you that you've been using drugs to numb, you'll never get 100% better.

## WHO IS MOST AT RISK FOR ADDICTION?

There are four primary components that make each of us more or less vulnerable to addiction:

**1. GENETIC PREDISPOSITION:** *Scientists will never find a single genetic trait that causes addiction, but they estimate that a person's genetics account for 40-60 percent of their risk. If you want to break a cycle of addiction, it is critical to learn and share your family history.*

*I was genetically predisposed through my mother (who was battling with her own addiction to heroin when she died) and her family. My father was open about my mother's addiction, but I was not closely connected with my mother's side of the family after her suicide. My father reasonably assumed that I would not turn to drugs or alcohol because of my* mother's horrific example; neither of us understood the full weight of my genetic background.

Since my kids have been able to communicate, I have talked to them about my experiences being addicted and taken them to my mom's grave site. They have attended my speaking engagements and support group meetings, as both a constant reminder of the consequences of choosing drugs and alcohol and the beauty created from continuous sobriety.

**2. EMOTIONAL TRAUMA:** Emotional pain and physical pain activate the same areas of our brains — the brain just doesn't distinguish between "hurt feelings" and "hurt bodies." Pain is one of the most powerful sensations that our brains can register; if something is too painful, our brains can quickly "rewire" in an attempt to keep us safe. That trauma-based rewiring can influence us to experience the world in constant response to that acute pain.

The emotional trauma of my mother's suicide affected me deeply, and made me even more vulnerable to addiction. My birth mom had a dysfunctional family environment that influenced her choice to abuse drugs and her eventual suicide. Many people who have faced severe trauma, though, never develop a drug or alcohol problem. My stepmother is a great example. She experienced extreme versions of many of the risk factors, but never succumbed to addiction or alcoholism. The real factor with trauma is how you learn and choose to cope with it.

**3. ENVIRONMENT:** *Good relationships and healthy, pleasurable surroundings stimulate the brain's reward path. Troubled relationships and places that make us feel bad, bored, sad, or stressed don't. If we don't find enough natural reward in the people we surround ourselves with, the places we go, and the things we do, we're more likely to try to stimulate our brains with risky behavior. This includes using drugs and alcohol, but also commonly unprotected sex, driving under the influence (every thirty minutes, someone is killed as a result of drinking and driving), and testing financial limits with activities like gambling and overspending.*

*I engaged in many risky behaviors, alienated my family and friends, disqualified myself from hockey (the thing I loved most), and spent much of my twenties shuttling between an apartment I'd made into a hovel or living out of my car. All in all, I created an environment where I was always increasingly vulnerable to the worst consequences of addiction.*

**4. CHOICES:** *We make cognizant choices to use drugs or alcohol. Obviously, these choices are influenced by the other three, but addiction is not deterministic. We participate.*

There are many, many other risk factors. There are large ones that intersect with each of these four primary components and affect huge swaths of the population, like low self-esteem. I also learn about more niche risk factors all the time. One that recently came across my radar is gastric bypass surgery. The low self-esteem that often leads people to develop overeating disorders, the alienation they felt while obese, and the actual medical and nutritional devastation the surgery wreaks on the body can all magnify the desire for drugs (especially amphetamines).

Addiction exists in all corners of our world. Risk factors don't discriminate. They are found across every demographic, every religion, economic stratum, race, and sexual orientation. We all exist on a spectrum of risk for drug and alcohol abuse. Being less at risk isn't a guarantee of sobriety, and having a high risk isn't an indicator of certain addiction. We are all part of vulnerable categories. That can be scary, but it can be liberating too. There is strength in understanding you are not alone.

We can't choose our genetic codes (although we can use the information we have about our family histories to guide our choices), we can't choose the pain we experienced in our pasts (although we can work to heal and grow), and we might not be able to snap our fingers and completely change our environments (though we will talk about the many things we can do to improve them). The most important factor is the one we control:

our choices.

The bottom line is that life often boils down to choices and consequences. Knowing that is a huge responsibility, but it helps us make choices that lead to the results we want: our best lives. No matter how many risk factors you face, you can embrace the endless opportunities that sobriety offers.

## IS SOMEONE REALLY AN ADDICT IF THEY HAVEN'T HIT ROCK BOTTOM?

"Rock bottom" and "addict" are both popular recovery terms that don't really fit into my mindset. I believe that anything is possible with sobriety, and I know that by living healthy, balanced, holistic lifestyles, we're capable of accomplishing more and feeling better than we ever would dream possible when we are using substances. Although some of us lose everything but our lives before we decide to get sober, many others chose sobriety before facing any serious, long-term consequences. Wherever you are in your life, whatever you are doing, you can always choose to get sober and start working towards not suffering.

Every step of recovery isn't going to be fun and easy, but making that first choice is amazing, something to be truly proud of. We don't need to concentrate on the wrong choices you made before—we need to celebrate the right choices you're making now. You'll be amazed how quickly you can stack them up! You'll discover the amazing person you are and build the life you want to live. You're going to be able to tackle whatever consequences you face as a strong, healthy person with a true understanding of your value and self-worth. Whether you're facing serious legal issues or have just noticed something beautiful in life you want to enjoy to the fullest, sobriety is an option within your grasp and begging to be chosen.

## HOW LONG DOES SOMEONE HAVE TO QUIT BEFORE THEY'RE SOBER?

By my early twenties, everyone was sick of me. My girlfriend was going to leave me; my family and most of my friends wouldn't even pick up my calls. My life, as crummy as I'd made it, was just about to collapse, and I couldn't handle it. I needed to do something to make them happy and get them back.

So, I stopped drinking.

I started stringing together one miserable day of forcing myself not to drink after another, and one month crawled by...then two...then eight...

And after nine of the worst months of my life, I quit quitting.

Pop quiz: Nine months is about 270 days. How many days was I sober?

Answer: ZERO.

Choosing not to drink and use drugs is NOT the same thing as choosing sobriety. It's an important part of sobriety, but it's not even close to the whole thing.

In the recovery community, forcing yourself not to drink when you really want to is commonly referred to as being a "dry drunk." Many people come to Racing for Recovery "dry." They're here because they're about to lose their jobs or their families, or they're trying to beat a drug charge or DUI, or the courts ordered them here. They can go through the program without any drugs or alcohol for weeks, months, or years—but that doesn't make them sober. Sadly, some clients leave us still just "dry."

You can't choose sobriety for your job or your family or anyone/anything else you love and are scared to lose. You can't build the foundation of sobriety on anything you can't control, and you can't control anything but your own choices. If you don't use substances because you don't want to face certain external consequences (or you want to gain some external reward), you're always betting on those things working out the way you want. Say that you're not going to drink because you don't want to be kicked out of school, or your mom promises to buy you a car if you stop using drugs. What happens when you graduate? What happens after those car keys are in your hand? In both of those examples, you "won"; what happens if you "lose" your external motivation? If it turns out that your mom can't afford the car or you flunk out, are you going to start using again, or are you going to focus on another consequence to base not using on? How many different bribes or threats are you going to run through? Not doing drugs but still wanting to do them is a bad place to be in; sooner or later, most people that try to live there permanently start using again.

Choosing not to drink or use drugs isn't a bad thing—it's a great thing! Not everyone chooses the whole sobriety package in one piece. Not using can be a good start. It can help you clear your thoughts and create space between your life and the substances you've been using. It can help you build stronger relationships and start healthy activities and good habits that make it easier to choose sobriety.

Choosing sobriety means choosing yourself. It means recognizing that choosing drugs and alcohol hurts you. If you're mourning and missing drugs and alcohol, you haven't chosen sobriety; you haven't chosen to care about the person you are and can be enough to feel fiercely protective. Choosing sobriety means choosing to take the first step to building yourself a life worth living.

I recently saw an interview with Steven Tyler from Aerosmith. I would love to work with him on a recovery level. Sure, I am a fan of his music, but that's not why. I feel like we could help him, as he indicated he struggles with

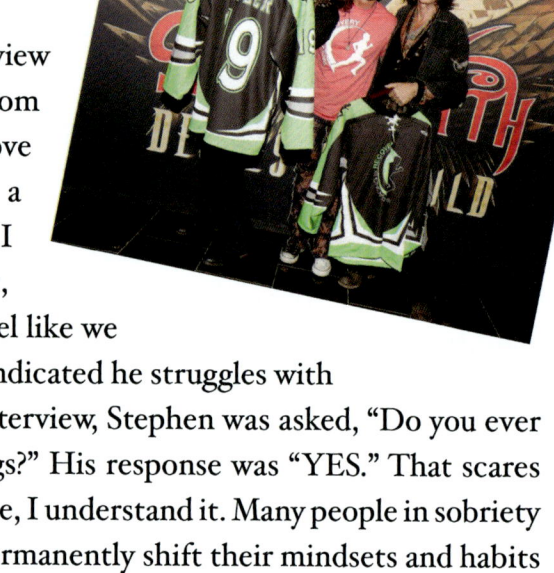

sobriety. During the interview, Stephen was asked, "Do you ever think about using drugs?" His response was "YES." That scares me, but at the same time, I understand it. Many people in sobriety aren't shown how to permanently shift their mindsets and habits to a place where you are so committed to how awesome you are that missing drugs is inconceivable.

People who are "dry" tend to spend a lot of time and energy thinking about why they still want to use because they "miss the high." Addiction is real and drugs have a powerful effect on your brain. Many people who have chosen sobriety still experience triggers or cravings for the drugs they once used. They can recognize that those aren't anything to be ashamed of or hide from. They're experiencing a brief reflex to pain. No one wants to be in pain. "Dry" and "missing the high" means you'd rather hide than deal with what's hurting you; choosing sobriety is realizing you deserve not to be in pain and committing to finding solutions in a balanced, holistic lifestyle.

## WHAT ABOUT MARIJUANA? WHAT ABOUT MEDICATIONS?

"Here," my friend said in a froggy voice, trying not to exhale.

I stared down at the bong he'd thrust towards me. I wasn't shocked. I knew the score when my buddies had picked me up. I'd sat in the van, chugging my fifth, and watched them go through the rituals of preparation, packing, and lighting it.

But I wanted no part in it. Weed was for stoners and dropouts and losers. I was an athlete. Getting high was one thing, but I didn't smoke drugs. I had standards.

I shrugged and took my first hit off a bong. I felt the smoke collect in my lungs, bringing some more shame, guilt, and disappointment along with it. It felt like a new low, a mile marker taking me further from the person I wanted to be.

That was in the autumn of my junior year of high school. By my senior year, I was packing my own bong along with my goalie mask and pads when I went off to practice every morning. By seven A.M., my buddies and I would be off the ice, in my car, and making our ways through a dime bag or so before classes started. Weed entered the rotation with Valium and alcohol that punctuated my days. It stayed in the rotation as I added more drugs (both type and quantity) into my daily grind over the next decade.

The crazy thing was that I never even liked pot. It made me feel lousy and paranoid. But I was deeply committed to self-destruction and rarely said 'no' to drugs, and marijuana, even then, was easy to come by.

Drugs, like every other element of culture, go through fads and phases of popularity. My drug use spanned from 1980 to 1993, the Reagan Revolution. It was an era between the hippies of the 60s and 70s and the Bill "Never Inhaled" Clinton presidency, and pot was not cool. Doctors weren't prescribing it, states weren't legalizing it, celebrities and CEOs weren't advocating for it.

The culture has changed now. In 2019, D.C. joined thirty-three other states to legalize cannabis for medical purposes. Eleven states have deemed it "recreational," giving it the same legal status as alcohol. There's a steady stream of public advocacy for it, extolling the virtues and parading out famous, successful users. We're all heavily bombarded with messages that pot is natural and fun and useful and the beautiful people are using it. Some of my colleagues in the wider recovery community even advocate for it as a treatment for substance abuse.

Understandably, I meet a lot of people who want to know if marijuana is a healthy alternative to other drugs.

It's a tricky subject to tackle, since pot is currently being touted as a cure-all for everything, from pain management to boredom. We're going to split the conversation into recreational use and medical use.

## RECREATIONAL MARIJUANA

I can be very clear on recreational use: Marijuana has no place in a balanced, holistic, sober, happy life. Sober people do not use drugs or alcohol recreationally.

Our culture promotes the idea that most people can drink responsibly and in moderation as a fun activity. More and more, we're getting the message that most people can use marijuana the same way. I'm not the guy who goes around telling people they have to live their lives the way I do—but I am telling you that is not part of choosing sobriety.

In a very real way, we all live inside our own heads. Our feelings, thoughts, and perceptions of the world are all very individual and brain-based. What you feel and experience is part of a complicated messaging system. When you are happy, that's because your brain is sending four chemicals through your reward system: dopamine, serotonin, oxytocin, and endorphin.

• Dopamine motivates us to do things, whether it's working on a big project or strapping on your shoes to run a race. If you're low on dopamine, you're going to be less motivated—you'll want to do the easy thing, even if it's not that great, rather than the harder thing that's way better.

• Serotonin makes us feel important and worthwhile. It's why looking back over the cool things we've accomplished feels so good. Try it right now—think about your last accomplishment. It doesn't have to be anything huge—did you make someone smile? Win a game? Find something you'd misplaced? The good feeling you get recalling that memory is serotonin-based. When you're low on serotonin, you feel like you're not worth much.

• Oxytocin makes us feel loved and helps us trust people. That feeling you get when you're wrapped in a good hug or you get a great gift is oxytocin. If you're low on oxytocin, you feel very isolated and alienated from other people.

• Endorphin makes us feel relaxed and gives us the message that all is right in the world. Your brain releases endorphin when you're exercising (that's the famous 'runner's high') or when you laugh hard. When you're low on endorphin, you're more sensitive to pain, both physically and emotionally.

Drugs don't make these chemicals—you do. Drugs are just a shortcut to trigger a rush of those chemicals that you are making.

A big part of the Racing for Recovery program is that we're trying to really do all the cool things we can and be the awesome people we want to be. We're earning those chemical rushes. We all tried

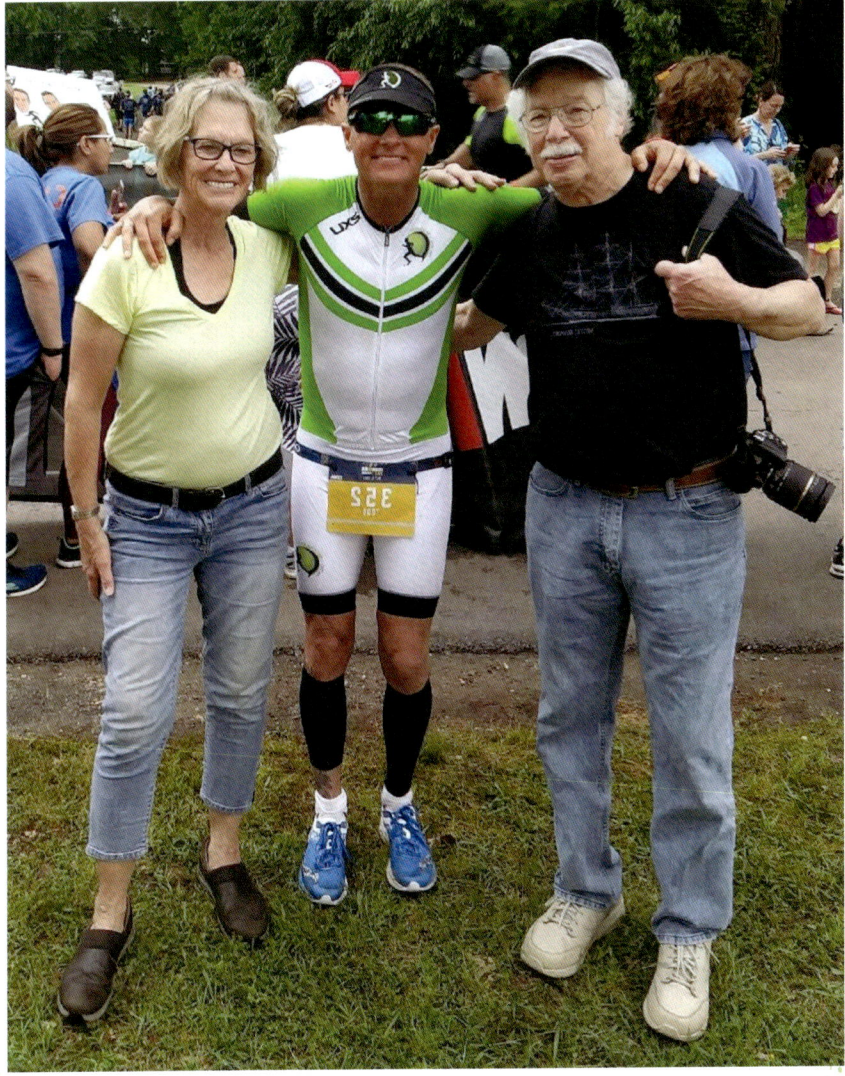

With my amazing parents at IRONMAN Virginia 70.3 2019

taking shortcuts before, and it didn't work for us. Pot and alcohol are made from plants, but that doesn't make their effects on our brains natural. Trust me, there's not enough drugs in this world to make you feel the way you do when you finish a race, when you're able to say, "I'm an IRONMAN!" There's no quick hit for getting an amazing hug in a relationship you worked really hard to build. Recreational drugs are cheap imitations of the complex, way better things you can be, do, and create. Choosing sobriety is about choosing yourself and all the things you can do instead of chemicals you can briefly trick your brain into releasing.

## MEDICAL MARIJUANA (AND OTHER MEDICINES)

I want to be clear up front: I am NOT a medical doctor. The perspective I'm going to share with you is from my experience and education as a counselor and as a person. Please talk to your doctor about any questions and concerns you have about medicines that you are prescribed, taking, and/or considering.

I'm not anti-medicine. It's pretty great to live in a world where I don't have to worry about chicken pox, polio, or the plague taking me out. I appreciate that my doctor doesn't pull out the leeches when I get an ear infection. It's nice not to wait around for lockjaw to set in if I get a cut.

Many of my clients come in with chronic pain (one of the conditions medical marijuana is prescribed for). An estimated 100 million Americans—one-third of the population—lives in chronic pain, meaning that they experience pain for more than twelve weeks straight. A lot of those people can manage their pain with treatments like physical therapy, meditation, and Tylenol. Others can't (or aren't presented with these alternatives), which is difficult. Chronic pain isn't well understood, and it's notoriously difficult for doctors to treat; they often prescribe highly addictive opioids to try and mask it. That has devastated many lives.

In a perfect world, all pain would be useful—we'd touch something hot, our brains would tell us that was hurting us, and we'd have a chance to stop before it hurt worse. When we brushed our burn against something, our brains would send us another pain message so that we'd protect that sensitive area and give it time to heal.

We don't live in a perfect world, and not all pain is useful. That sucks, and I wish it was different. I also wish I could write a blank check for whatever drugs people in chronic pain could use to mask it, but I can't. I see too many people at Racing for Recovery who are dealing with not only chronic pain, but lives destroyed by the painkillers that were prescribed by doctors to try to help with it.

The drugs that can mask pain, from opioids to marijuana, work through some combination of dulling the receptors in the brain that are registering that something hurts, flooding the brain with endorphin, and making the brain more receptive to endorphin. The problem is that we can only trick our brains with these floods for a little while before they get used to it. Without any other treatment, those pain signals keep coming. Our brains reset to consider that chemically-induced flood of endorphin as the new normal, and they rewire to let those pain messages get through. Then we need more medicines and stronger doses to get results. That's called 'tolerance.'

Marijuana has also entered the conversations I have with clients about psychiatric medications. It is prescribed for anxiety, depression, and PTSD, three diagnoses that many people with addictions battle. Every statistic you can find will tell you that there's a strong link between mental health and addiction. In my experience, that link is universal: No one can be mentally healthy and have an addiction. Most of the people that I meet, myself included, chose to use drugs to mask emotional trauma. Those who didn't (who usually started using drugs prescribed for pain) developed emotional trauma as their choice to continue using drugs started tearing through their lives, relationships, and senses of self worth.

It's no secret that our society has a mental health crisis. There's a psychiatric "bible" that's updated and published every so often, the Diagnostic and Statistical Manual of Mental Disorders (DSM). Whenever a new version comes out, it makes

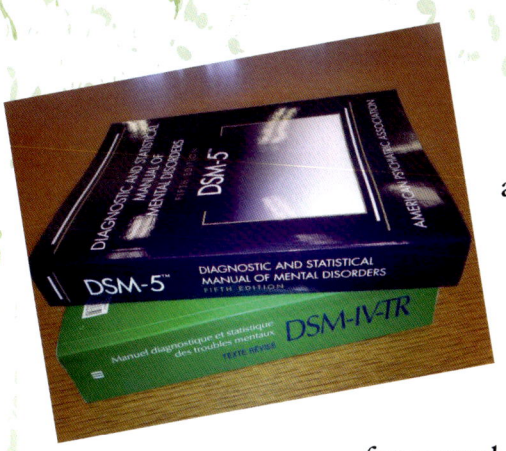

a lot of news, because it's the officially recognized source of every mental disorder diagnosis. It gives us the names, classifications, and checklists of symptoms for mental health concerns, and sets the official boundaries for what is considered "normal" and what is considered "pathological." Beyond its use in treating individuals, it's a fascinating snapshot of what we believe mental health looks like at any given time. Homosexuality was considered a mental disorder until 1973! The word "addiction" doesn't appear in the newest version at all!

There's a pretty wide split between the way that doctors make psychiatric diagnoses and most modern medical diagnoses. If you have a sore throat, the doctor will take a close look at it, then order a bacterial culture (strep test), or blood samples for testing, or an x-ray, etc. There are no bacterial cultures, blood tests, or x-rays when you go to a doctor because you are sad, scared, or stressed (though there are now some "biomarkers" used to diagnose sleep disorders). Instead, they ask you for descriptions of how you're feeling and how that's affecting your life, and they compare your answers to the checklists in the DSM to diagnose you.

I've seen how those diagnoses can be hard on a person who is already struggling with emotional issues. Being told you have strep throat usually isn't too scary, because a few days of medicine can almost always clear it up. You're not permanently "strep-throated." But many medical diagnoses can affect the rest of your life. When you're diagnosed with cancer, even if your treatment is very successful and there are no signs of cancer left in your body, most doctors won't say that you're "cured"—they'll say you're "in remission." Once you're diagnosed with diabetes, even if every other blood test for the rest of your life shows balanced glucose levels, you're still considered "in remission." When someone is diagnosed with something like ADD or an anxiety disorder, most people don't understand that's a snapshot of how their brains are working at one moment in time—a snapshot that can shift and change drastically through the course of your life. Like labeling addiction as a disease, these diagnoses can seem permanent and out of our control.

In 2013, when the DSM-5 came out, some people estimated that the edits that had been made could classify almost 50% of the population as "pathological."

Nearly 70% of people in the United States take some type of prescribed drugs; the second most common prescription is for anti-depressants, and the third is opioids. Almost half of Americans twelve and older take prescription pain relievers, tranquilizers, sedatives, or stimulants. Over 500,000 kids are currently on antidepressant medications, and over 19,000 of them are under the age of five. And every year, those numbers rise.

Guys, something is terribly wrong.

I'm certainly not alone in believing that drugs are being over-prescribed. A huge part of the problem is that we're focused more on making our problems (or sometimes just our kids themselves) "manageable" than addressing the root issue.

As a clinician, when clients tell me they feel they need to rely on drugs, whether those drugs are legally prescribed or not, I want to understand WHY. It is more important to me to get to the bottom of the issue. Masking a problem leads to misery and more problems; masking it with medical marijuana (even though it's a plant) still isn't a solution. If you're medicating to manage, rather than heal, it doesn't matter whether you're self-medicating or you've got a prescription—you're not actually dealing with the underlying issue.

I'm not writing off psychiatric medications when there is a critical need and they are used as part of the therapeutic process. Getting to that WHY is hard work that takes clear thinking, the ability to confront the root of your pain, and a real belief that you can get better. When I'm working with people who are on medications, I suggest they talk to their prescribing doctors about how those medications affect their emotions and thoughts; if they choose to work towards tapering their doses or stopping, that's great. Either way, I want to help people become the best versions of themselves, and many are surprised by how powerfully the balanced, holistic Racing for Recovery life changes their minds and bodies. Learning the ways that you can rely on your own awesome self is empowering.

Marijuana and prescription medications become more accessible every day. The chances that you'll be offered these drugs is nearly the same as the chances that you'll have the opportunity to drink—100%. The picture of happy, beautiful, successful people using pot that society seems to be pushing looks oddly identical to old cigarette advertisements (another all-natural plant that is NOT healthy). You're not being sold happiness—you're being sold on the idea that you're not enough. People make obscene profits off of making you feel like you're not good enough without their product, and the pharmaceutical, alcohol, and marijuana markets aren't being run by not-for-profits. Choosing sobriety is telling those people that who you are and what you can do is way more interesting than shoveling over your money, time, and talents to them.

## SIX PHASE CYCLE OF ADDICTION

**ACTING OUT:** Under stress and without better coping mechanisms, an individual struggling with addiction will cause trouble or turn to the substances they've used to alleviate stress in the past.

**REGRET:** The individual feels badly about acting out, but cannot change the past, which causes pain and self-loathing.

**RECONSTITUTION:** The individual tries to put their life back together and "do the right thing" to alleviate their regret. This is often confused for recovery.

**DORMANT:** The individual tries to replace their addiction with some other form of high or exhaust themselves to the point of distraction.

**TRIGGER:** The individual encounters internal and external factors that make them want to choose drugs and alcohol.

**PREPARATION:** The individual has chosen sobriety, is doing the work to create a life free of addiction, and living with inner peace and tranquility.

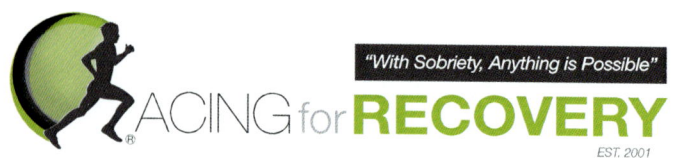
"With Sobriety, Anything is Possible"

RACING for RECOVERY

EST. 2001

# CHOOSE HEALING

Once you choose sobriety, you face all the reasons you started drinking and drugging in the first place. No one chooses drugs because everything is going great in their lives—they do it to treat some pain that they don't have the skills to face alone. Drugs and alcohol act as Band-Aids to some pain, but underneath, the wound doesn't heal—and the consequences of masking that pain, rather than choosing to heal, just creates more trauma.

Healing your wounds, whether they are physical or mental, is a critical part of creating a happy, balanced life. Learning why you act and feel the way you do can help you find new ways to face your problems, and caring for your body and health will give you the strength you need.

## HOW DO I CURE MY TRAUMA?

Meet Frank, Hazel, and Gene:

One day, their bowl gets knocked off the ledge. Their world is literally flipped upside down. That is the traumatic incident.

Gene was asleep, and he fell right into a sink full of water. He experiences the traumatic incident as a minor inconvenience, swims away, and never thinks much of it again. Frank and Hazel fall to the floor, and Frank breaks a flipper. He experiences the traumatic incident as painful and scary, but he does not make any larger connections between this event and how the world operates. Once his flipper heals, he does not often consider the traumatic event. Hazel is physically unharmed, but it was the first time she'd truly comprehended that the bowl was capable of moving. Her brain, which was rapidly firing out powerful pain, panic, and stress signals during the traumatic event, processes these changes to her perception as really important for survival.

All three fish were involved in the same traumatic incident, but their bodies and minds absorbed the impact in very different ways. Gene does not carry any trauma. Frank carries physical trauma, but it doesn't sound like he's registered emotional trauma.

Hazel carries no physical trauma, but she does carry emotional trauma. The traumatic event significantly reshaped the way her brain understands and processes the world. She now lives with the understanding that fishbowls can be upended, that she does not control it, and that she experiences upended fishbowls as scary and painful. The ways this trauma changes how she feels and reacts to the world depend on what coping mechanisms she had before the traumatic incident and which ones she learns afterwards.

We're usually not aware of it, but our brains are constantly comparing what is currently happening around us to what has happened to us in the past. If something in your situation now resembles a memory, your brain will skim through that memory for helpful information (the best choices we can make and the consequences we can expect). If that memory is attached to intense emotions, you will experience those emotions all over again.

Most people who struggle with addiction have childhood traumas. Trauma that you experience when you are younger can be particularly damaging because...

**1) YOU DO NOT HAVE AS MANY EMOTIONAL RESPONSES TO CHOOSE FROM WHEN THE TRAUMATIC EVENT OCCURS.** We're not born with many ways to deal with pain, and certainly not emotional pain. We're not actually born with emotions at all! As newborns, we have two states of being: pleasant and unpleasant. If something is unpleasant, we cry. That's it, end of coping mechanisms.

As we experience more of the world, we start to develop emotions in response. Our first three are happy, angry, and fearful. It takes us a long time to develop a sophisticated sense of impulse control, much less internal regulation. Our emotions are "bigger" when we're young because we don't have as many to choose from. A two-year-old who doesn't get the cereal he wants hasn't developed "a little disappointed" as an emotion yet—the emotional response he has available is anger, which is why you get those intense temper tantrums.

**2) YOU HAVE A LIMITED NUMBER OF EXPERIENCES TO COMPARE THE TRAUMATIC EVENT TO.** This is not to downplay the severity of your traumatic incident! Remember, your brain is always scanning your past memories to get information to help you right now. The less memories that you have built up to scan, the more situations that each will be the best information you have available. For example, say you wake up and it's snowing. If it's the second time you've seen snow, your brain will rely on the only memory of snow you've got for information. If you've seen 100 snowstorms, your brain will look through the ones that most resemble this one for the best information. If you burn yourself on the stove the first time you touch it, the fact that the stove can hurt you will be the only information you have on it. If you've cooked a bunch of meals before you get your first burn, the knowledge that the stove can hurt you will be balanced with the knowledge that you can also make delicious things with it and that it won't always burn you.

**3) WE REALLY HATE THE IDEA THAT THERE ARE THINGS WE CAN'T CONTROL.** No matter how old you are, the knowledge that there are things you can't control is really painful—it's scary! To move through the world in a healthy way, we have to be able to balance the idea that there are things outside of our control with our motivations. Our brains will do a lot to try to protect us from the idea that painful things can happen that we won't have a say in—including convince us that we were to blame. If we think it's our fault that the traumatic incident occurred, we think that means that we can control painful things from happening in the future. That type of thinking is particularly damaging when you haven't had the chance yet to build a sense of self-worth.

Say that you're walking out the door and a bird swoops down in your face. Your brain hates the idea that sometimes birds will swoop, and it will look for a thing that you did "wrong," so that you can control it happening again. If you've already accomplished things in life, you know that you can't be all bad and wrong, so you'll tie your sense of control to a small thing—oh man, it must be because I wore a yellow shirt! Now, all you have to do is stay away from yellow shirts. It's not true, but it helps you walk out the door in the future without being in constant fear of birds.

If you haven't had a chance yet to accomplish many things in life and build your sense of self-worth, you are just left with the idea that being you is the thing you did wrong, the thing you need to not do in the future to stop bad things from happening.

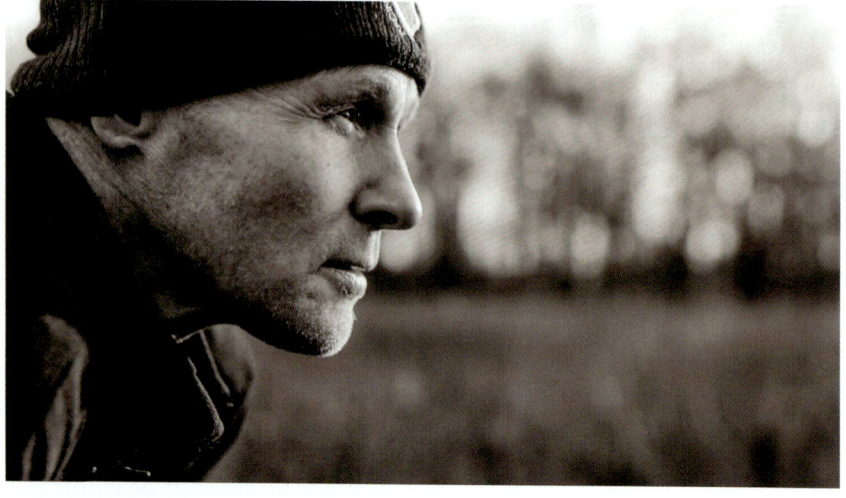

## SO ABOUT THAT CURE...

The hard truth is that the healing process for emotional trauma never ends. There's no "cure," because it stems from a painful incident in the past (which you cannot change) and an acute knowledge that painful things happen in the world that you cannot control (which is correct). When something happens, emotionally or in your environment, that your brain interprets as related to this traumatic event, it will recall the same painful emotions—remember, it's hardwired into you as an "important survival lesson." Choosing to heal from trauma is about learning new coping mechanisms and examining your understanding of the traumatic event. You cannot cure trauma, but you can radically change your relationship with it.

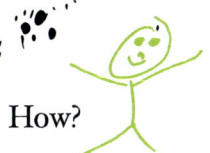

How?

**DEVELOP MORE AND BETTER COPING SKILLS:** When we have strong feelings of fear and anger, the coping mechanisms we naturally build up are based in defense and shame, which lead to self-destruction. When you self-medicate with drugs and alcohol, that's an example of a coping skill—just not a good one. We try to manage these traumas from the outside, try to consume something that will make it better. We need to focus inward first, to understand and heal, then utilize outside things to enhance the self-betterment that's already taking place. It is important to develop a variety of coping skills—more skills create better results. Every choice that we discuss in this book is an example of a coping skill; the more good choices you make, the more good coping skills you will rack up.

**RECOGNIZE THAT YOUR TRAUMATIC EMOTIONS ARE TEMPORARY:** When traumatic emotions arise, they are just as intense as they've always been. Accept the fact that you will sometimes have these emotions, but that they are not permanent, and that you can do so much to heal. The danger is when we believe there is no end to our grief. As you develop your strength, better coping mechanisms, and your balanced holistic lifestyle, they will be farther and farther apart, and you'll be able to pull yourself out of these mental ruts quickly.

**GET OVER GETTING OVER IT:** My mother committed suicide

almost fifty years ago, and it still affects me. *For years, I would fight it—this should not bother me! I don't even remember my mom. Why is this still haunting me? Why can't I get over it? What's wrong with me?!?!*

Ugh—"get over it" might be the dumbest advice that we're given and give ourselves in relationship to our pain. **Trauma is *REAL!*** Like, as physically real as the book you're holding (or tablet, computer, phone—you know what I mean, wiseguy). You can't see it happening, but it's a provable series of chemical reactions wiggling through your entire nervous system. Without a time machine (don't try this at home) or a lobotomy (DON'T TRY THIS AT HOME!), every moment of your history is what it is. It's part of what makes you who you are (and, reminder, you're awesome).

Realizing that I wasn't "doing healing wrong" was a huge relief, and it opened up my world so that I could heal the things that were actually broken. Anybody who's gone through anything horrible can stop self-destructing and start to heal as you start living a full life.

The people who tell you to get over it aren't bad or even trying to hurt you. Some of them probably really love you, and they're struggling with the fact they can't help you. When you hear them tell you to get over it, realize that what they are saying is that they are frustrated that they can't make your pain go away. Other people are expressing the fact that they cannot emotionally handle the fact that trauma and pain exist. They have problems with the idea that things exist outside of their own control. Realize that they might be saying, "Get over it!" at you, but they're really talking to themselves.

Either way, now you know better. Stop saying it to yourself and don't say it to other people!

**DON'T COMPARE YOUR TRAUMA:** When you hurt, it's natural to look around and try to figure out why other people don't. Sometimes this is useful, like when you're able to learn a new coping mechanism. But your trauma is as individual as your fingerprints, because it's based in your experiences and your history. It's not useful to compare it with someone else's. You can't judge anyone else's trauma, and they can't judge yours.

It's tough when your trauma is based in an event similar to or that you even shared with others, like growing up in an abusive household with other siblings. You might all be affected differently, but none of you are "wrong." Think back to Frank, Hazel, and Gene. They were all involved in the same traumatic incident, but

Gene was fine—that didn't make Frank's flipper any less broken! The way that it affected Hazel was just as real and just as "valid." You can't dismiss how someone else feels, even if it seems like they are being dramatic or exaggerating their experiences, and they can't dismiss yours.

**IDENTIFY YOUR TRIGGERS:**
Start paying attention to the things that make you vulnerable and susceptible to your pain, and the things that you choose to manage those. For me, when I don't exercise, I 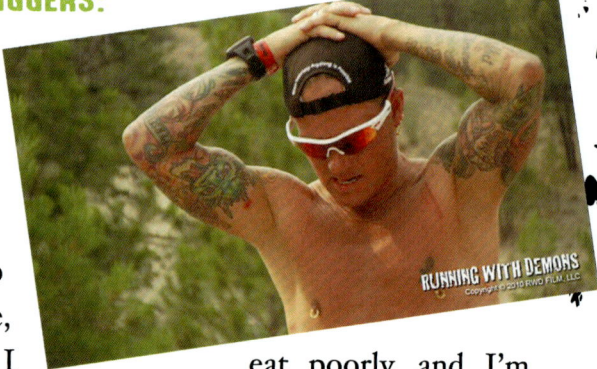 eat poorly, and I'm tired, it's easier for me to slip into my dark thought patterns. Even though our bodies need them to recover and heal, it's hard for me to have off-days from swimming, biking, and running. Without that endorphin rush, it's easy for me start entertaining truly miserable ideas about myself. Since I know off-days are a trigger for me, I'll do things to make sure my schedule for that day is very active—that it is not a day that I have to sit behind a desk for long stretches of time, a day where I am interacting with people who have energy and positivity that I can engage with.

**VISUALIZE THE POSSIBILITIES:** If you are compelled to react in

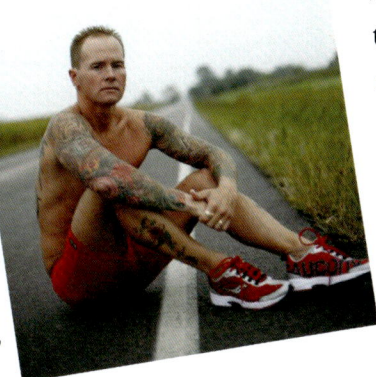

ways you're not proud of when you're triggered, practice visualizing the reactions and good decisions you'd rather make when you are in an untriggered, safe time and place. It's like asking the best, wisest version of you for advice on how to handle situations. It also preps your brain to realize there's another option when you're triggered again. You know how you're always scanning your memory? Well, in that scan, your brain doesn't distinguish between a memory that actually happened and a story you get really into telling yourself. You're giving yourself more data and better data points to consider when you're facing something you find tough. You can rack up the mental strength and benefits of making the right choices before you even face a situation—think about how cool that is!

**TALK, TALK, TALK:** When something happens that stimulates us, whether it's watching a horror movie or playing a great game, we process things better when we express them to others. Using drugs and alcohol is a way of hiding from that processing. Choosing to tell your story, over and over and over, as many times as you need to and in as much detail, helps you start to understand it in new ways and emotionally process it through every new coping mechanism you acquire. It helps you identify patterns of thinking and behaviors that hurt you. It helps you reason through feelings of shame, blame, and worthlessness. You can learn new perspectives from people who love and care about you, and you can even help other people who have traumatic emotions they still need to process.

Find as many ways as you can express yourself and tell your story. Draw a comic! Play music! Write a book!!

Dave Rude from TESLA
He did the instrumental soundtrack for Running with Demons

**SEEK HELP:** There are many resources for professional help in your communities, but they sometimes seem invisible unless you actively search them out. Ask your school, work, religious group, town, friends, and family what type of support options exist. Let people help you.

I know what it's like to feel like your pain is too much, like no one could possibly help, like anyone you could open up to would hate you if they really knew you, and like you're completely alone in this. It's awful. But I was wrong, and you are too. I'm one of those people in your community, and I can't tell you how much you mean to me. Helping you isn't a burden—it is an **AMAZING PRIVILEGE,** a **GIFT** that I work really hard to deserve. You make me better; let me (and the many people like me) return the favor.

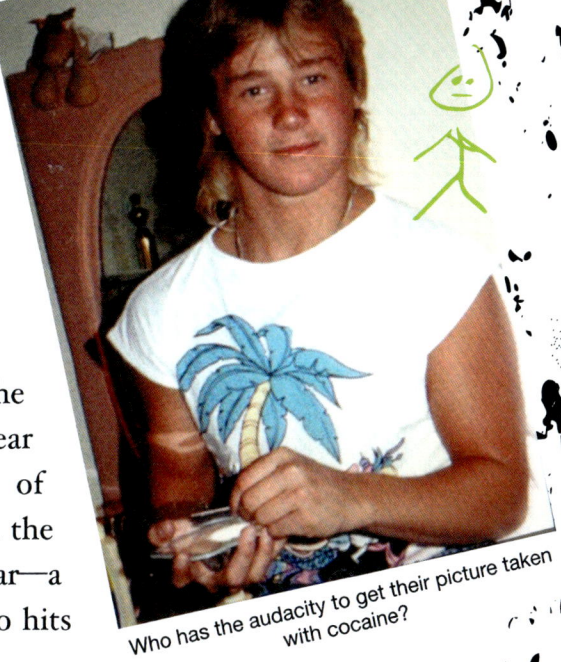

Who has the audacity to get their picture taken with cocaine?

## AM I WEAK?

I had my first drink the summer before freshman year of high school—a few sips of beer. I had my second drink the first weekend of freshman year—a fifth of Jack Daniels and two hits of speed.

Go big or go home, right? (I definitely should have chosen to go home.)

I drank heavily every weekend for the first two years of high school, and the amount and frequency only increased from there. I kept choosing drugs and alcohol, over and over again, and the consequences kept getting more severe—legal, emotional, physical, academic, and social.

Six years after that first drink, I sat alone on the sand at Cocoa Beach, Florida, hunched over a bottle of cheap vodka, trying to keep the rain off my face. I had been kicked off my hockey team, kicked out of school, kicked out of my parents' house.

I was looking at an eight-year prison term for receiving stolen property. I was homeless, addicted, and living in my car. I'd lost everything—my spirit, friends, faith, hope, willingness to succeed. **EVERYTHING**. I just kept asking myself, How did I end up here? I was going to be a pro hockey player. I drank until I passed out underneath an air conditioner in the window of some fleabag motel.

Merry Christmas.

I woke up to the blazing Florida sunshine, sicker than a dog. I realized my necklace had been torn off and stolen.

I found the card my parents had sent me: "Remember Christmas past..." I opened it, hoping against hope for some cash. "Because this is your Christmas present." There was a picture of an elf holding a candle—that was it.

Seemed about right.

Something about that punishing sun pierced through my mental fog—just enough to give me the vaguest idea that this didn't have to be my life. I didn't have to drink myself into an oblivion...

The devastation on my low self-worth was brutal, because I didn't think I was ready to make that choice. I didn't think I deserved to make that choice. It took me another seven years to choose sobriety.

## DOES THAT MAKE ME WEAK?

Addiction is a response to the core issue of trauma. We are hurting people who do not know how to handle that pain. It is normal to not want to hurt. It is normal to want pain to stop. In order to deal with it, we choose to self-medicate with drugs or alcohol. Unfortunately, this method of coping leads to more poor choices and unwanted consequences. It is a vicious cycle of pain, substance abuse, grief, then more pain.

Pain and trauma cause low self-worth. Low self-worth keeps us from pursuing the things that we want and healthy relationships. It keeps us from living our purpose and enjoying life.

I did drugs and drank because I did not feel right emotionally. I was searching for a way to destroy myself because I had no self-worth.

## DOES THAT MAKE ME WEAK?

I abandoned myself with drugs, the ultimate expression of self-loathing for somebody with abandonment issues. I truly believed that everybody else had done it, everybody else hated me enough to abandon me, and I hated myself enough to abandon myself. That self-loathing was so deeply ingrained in me that it outlasted my addiction. I look back now on the Running with Demons documentary, and realize that, even sixteen years sober, even as an IRONMAN many times over, with every other gift I had, I still hated myself so much that I spent a lot of time living in constant grief.

## DOES THAT MAKE ME WEAK?

Sorry to keep asking, it's just...well, your question doesn't make sense.

### PEOPLE AREN'T WEAK.

People can make weak choices. We can weaken our situations, our bodies, and our lives. We can be overwhelmed and incredibly hurt. We can have low self-esteem. We can feel very broken. But as long as we are alive, we have the potential to heal, grow, and build strong, balanced, healthy lives. Choosing to heal means choosing to understand that you are always strong, that you always have incredible value, because you always have the ability to make strong choices.

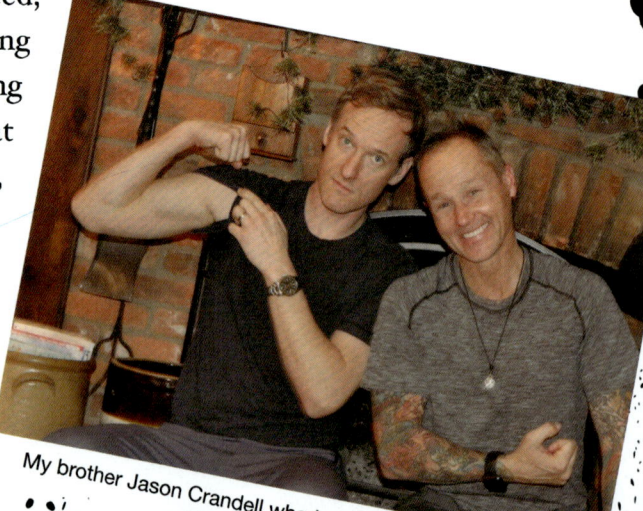

My brother Jason Crandell who I admire and respect greatly

It doesn't matter if your last choice was weak—if your last million choices were weak. You can make your next choice a strong one, and the one after that, and the one after that.

I wasn't weak, sitting on that beach when I was nineteen. Everything I've built in life, I built from that point, and many dark points afterwards. Even when I couldn't see it—even when no one could see it—I was the strongest dude on Earth. I thought I'd thrown everything away, but I had more potential than I could use in a lifetime or two or three.

But this isn't really about me, is it?

## SO...ARE YOU WEAK?

You're reading this sentence, which means you're alive. Which means you are stronger than you can even comprehend. I hope you make the next choice a strong one, because you're going to start stacking up the benefits quickly. They're going to be awesome, and I can't wait to hear about them.

Finding self-worth starts with not doing self-destructive things. The only way to find what we are searching for is to stop abusing ourselves and start making strong choices.

**FROM ONE OF THE STRONGEST DUDES IN THE WORLD TO ANOTHER? CHOOSE TO HEAL. CHOOSE TO BUILD A LIFE AS STRONG AND INCREDIBLE AS YOU ARE.**

So, here's your brain:

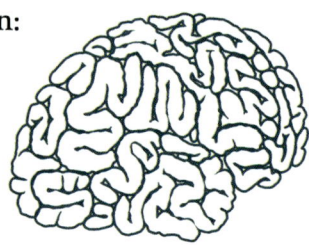

 It rewires itself all the time based off what you're experiencing. One of the things that can rewire a brain are powerful emotions—particularly pain. When you experience emotional trauma, your brain processes it as extreme pain, both acute and chronic. That pain affects how your brain is wired, which affects how you experience and react to the world.

Here's another view of your brain:

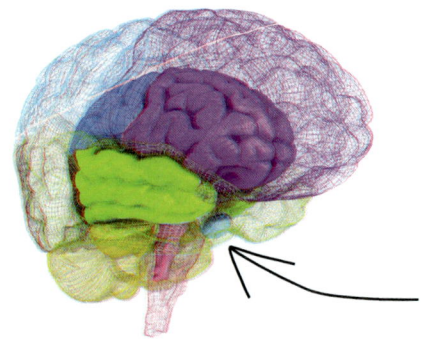

AMYGDALA

In really simplified terms, the amygdala is where your emotions are centered. It preps you for fight or flight. The frontal lobes help you decide between the two. The most functional way for your brain to process emotions and impulses is for these two parts to work together. When you're highly emotional, the frontal lobes can stop working properly, and the amygdala takes charge. That makes it much harder to control your emotions—and you lose it. If your brain has rewired around trauma, your frontal lobes can shut down even easier.

I used to lose it a lot. I didn't understand my anger was really pain—I felt rage, and I felt it (and acted on it) pretty frequently. I was always getting into fights.

Some of them were easy for me to justify, like beating up the guys who bullied me. My sophomore year, I was bullied relentlessly by one kid named Sean. He just tormented me daily—before, during, and after my last period gym class. (I had no idea what Sean's problem was until years later. He was in the audience at a local rehab center for one of my first talks. Afterward, he came up and told me he'd bullied me because he was jealous.)

I was scared to death of Sean (and weirdly admired him). He was tough and he had a nice Camaro. He would blast Motley Crue. He kept telling everyone he was going to fight me in the parking lot after school. The stares and jeers were bad, but the repetition of the threat was the worst part—I always had to wonder if today was the day. I was scared, but I never let on.

The last day of school, he followed me out to the parking lot, taunting me and calling me names the whole way. I ignored him until he shoved me from behind.

That was it.

I turned around and swung my fist along with my body. My built-up fears were released into rage and fury. My mind was surprisingly quiet and the scene unfolded almost as if it were in slow motion. Hundreds of kids watched.

The principal and some teachers came out, and one administrator grabbed me. In my fury, I accidentally landed a left punch to his stomach before I returned to letting this kid know never to mess with me again.

I was suspended from school and could not take my scheduled exams, but I got permission to take them the following week (during summer break), in the principal's office. That turned out well for me, because I had all of the answers by then. I made sure not to do too well. That would have raised a red flag.

A year later, a senior named Greg felt like he needed to confront me. He was one of the burnouts, who smoked and loitered outside the school in the smoking area (yes, there really was a smoking area at school), and every day for months, I sat in my American Literature class while he pantomimed beating me up.

One day, after the bell rang, I walked out of my class and to my locker. Greg walked in from the smoking area and stood right behind me, trying to get me to instigate the fight. I didn't. I opened my locker, and Greg slammed it on my left arm, cutting me on the top of my bicep just below my shoulder.

Greg was intimidating, with his black leather jacket, jeans, boots, etc. I was afraid when he slammed the locker door on me, but again, my inner rage roared. I stopped thinking, my mind went silent, and I beat him up good. Kids stood all around as I pulled his jacket over his head (kind of a hockey fight move) and threw punches left and right at his face until he had enough. The teachers broke us up, and I was escorted to the principal's office, where I was handed another suspension notice.

I didn't just take care of my own bullies. Senior year, my friend Bill told me he'd been beaten up by a couple of older guys. We drove over to one guy's house late at night and I stood on the front porch and rang the doorbell.

The boy's father opened the door and asked what we were doing there so late. I made up some story, and when his son came downstairs, I asked him to come outside and explain to me how my friend's face had gotten beaten so badly.

I could see this kid's fear as he told me, "Well, one thing led to another, and, oh well, I kinda guess I hurt him a little bit."

I paused for a moment and then, very calmly and coolly, said to him, "Well, I guess some things are about to get outta hand here as well."

I dragged this kid out into the front yard and physically pummeled him in front of his own father.

I got my friend Bill and we left. That was that. In my drunken, drugged-out, distorted mind, I thought I was showing my loyalty as a friend.

There were the fights I brought upon myself, like when my parents left town and left Grandma (who had no idea I was a drug addict) in charge.

I was sitting between two girls in the front seat of the car as we headed to McDonald's on a Friday night. As we rolled into the drive-thru, I spotted the girls' boyfriends in the parking lot. When we made eye contact, I put an arm around each of them and smirked.

The boys began yelling at me as the car stopped, and while the girls got their food, I got out of the car and walked up to their boyfriends. They grabbed me and pushed me up against the cement wall, but onlookers called the cops before anything could really happen.

The boys (one of whom was a police officer's son) got in a blue Trans Am and took off. I immediately found a friend and got in his car. He and I pursued them through the streets of Sylvania. We followed them for a few miles, flashing the headlights at them to pull over and continue what we'd started. Once they pulled into a local carryout and parked, I leaped out of the car before it stopped and ran over to the passenger's door.

I beat the kid in the passenger's seat badly. Then I walked over to the driver's side; this kid was trying to hold the door shut, but the window was down. I started punching him through the window until he let go of the door. When I opened the door, he fell out of the car and landed on the pavement. I got over him and kept punching him.

I heard someone yell, "I think he has had enough."

My friend said, "TC, you are going to kill that kid. STOP."

I gave him one final kick to the head (which I later found out put him in the hospital for several days). By this time, the owner of the carryout came out and said he was calling the police. We took off.

I was covered in blood. When I went home later that night, my grandma saw me and I told her what had happened.

My family wasn't shocked by my violence. My dad was always afraid my anger would land me in jail; thank God I didn't. One time, my grandmother taped a drunken conversation with me about my mom. The next day, when I was told she'd taped my words, I became extremely angry. I was embarrassed of how I felt, and more embarrassed when my grandma told me she was worried about me because "the venom I had towards my mother was frightening. My mom had been dead for most of my life, and I felt like I should have been over it and unaffected.

I would go to my mom's graveside and spit on it. Several times, I dumped beer or whiskey on it. I smashed empty beer bottles on it, and one time, I was told I tried to piss on it, but my friend stopped me.

That venom didn't disappear after I got sober. One time, my wife made me take flowers to her grave on Mother's Day. I just drove past her grave, threw the flowers out the window, and kept driving. My wife made me get out and place them on her grave nicely.

I wasn't ever really some tough guy. I was hurt, and instead of dealing with that pain, I chose to try to numb myself with drugs and alcohol. Even when I'd chosen sobriety, I didn't always choose to work on my healing. I stopped swinging my fists at people, but

I was still choosing to take my rage out on others.

My brain was reacting to trauma, but I was in charge. I made choices, over and over again, to continue acting on these impulses, to not seek help, to not find better solutions. Now, I have developed coping mechanisms to help me make better choices. I work through problems. I have taken a full inventory of my triggers, the things that could set me off, and I make an effort to avoid these situations and to take time to process, rather than just react. I practice a balance, healthy, holistic lifestyle that includes yoga and daily exercise.

I pay close attention to my mental diet. Who you talk to, what you watch, what you listen to, what you think and say, the conversations you let yourself have and the reactions that you allow yourself to have are all connected. Everything that you process is brain-food. It affects how you heal and how you grow and who you are becoming every day. Choose to mentally feed yourself positive, helpful things, and you'll get healthier and better able to control your emotions and your reactions. There are people who will pay attention to the nutrition in every bite of food they take, but mentally feed themselves hateful, negative, destructive things. It's worse than mental fast-food—it's a diet of rotting garbage, and it makes people very, very sick.

Part of your brain might be suggesting you lash out, but it's still your choice whether you're going to follow through. We can choose to consciously rewire our brains, the same way that they can be rewired by strong emotions. Repeated behavior creates habits, which can be difficult to break (and won't usually go away on their own). You have the power to create new habits, applying the same intensity and dedication to choosing better impulses that can overpower the old ones. Visualize your life the way you want it to be. This is a powerful way to rewire your brain, because your hippocampus doesn't distinguish between experiencing something and merely visualizing it. If you visualize, you can create the habits you want.

When we allow trauma to fester and deepen, we have less control over our emotions, and we act against what we know is right and unlike the people we want to be. Stop self-destructing, stop punishing yourself for mistakes, and start learning from them.

Fighting, arguing, and intense emotional grief create more unhappiness. By making healthy choices on a daily basis, you will rewire your brain to experience more feelings of contentment, optimism, joy, tranquility, and peace. Implement a balanced holistic lifestyle with proper nutrition, exercise, spirituality, education, family and peer support, and service, and you'll be amazed how much better you feel and how much easier it is to make better choices.

## AM I A BAD PERSON?

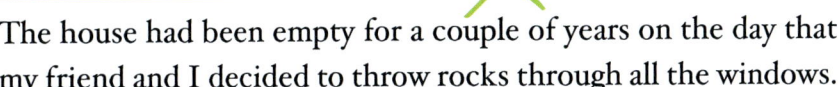

The house had been empty for a couple of years on the day that my friend and I decided to throw rocks through all the windows.

I can't remember why it seemed like a good idea. The sound of all that glass shattering was pretty cool, I guess, and I knew I could get away with it.

We went to school with a girl named Janet from a very low-income family. She had to shower in the gym, she didn't have many outfits, and she never had as much food as the rest of us did. It bothered me a lot, and I wasn't sure what to do about it, which bothered me even more.

Years later, I learned that Janet's family had lived in that vacant house I'd vandalized.

On one hand, I was destructive and often thoughtless. On the other, I cared about Janet and her family. When I discovered that she and her family had lived in that house, I was filled with empathy and remorse. The consequences of that simple act of senseless vandalism expanded my ability to feel for and understand others in ways I utilize now every day as a clinician to help people improve their lives.

People tend to group together based on particular qualities. That makes sense sometimes—if you really want to play soccer, you're going to be happier joining a soccer team than taking a drawing class and hoping they want to play soccer with you. Unfortunately, once we establish ourselves in groups, it's easy to slip into an "us versus them" mentality—what social psychologists call "ingroup" and "outgroup." The people in the outgroup—all those "thems"—seem weird to you. You can't really understand what makes them tick. Ingrouping and outgrouping can get really ugly very quickly, because it is easy for an inability to empathize to turn into mistrust, fear, and even hatred of your outgroup.

Growing up, I hated to see kids excluded. I was outgoing and popular, but it was easy for me to empathize with classmates who didn't seem very confident—because deep down, I didn't feel very good about myself either. I'll never forget Steve, the smartest kid in class. He got bullied a lot and he was afraid to be at school. I felt bad for him, so I moved his desk near mine, so nobody would mess with him.

I wasn't immune to outgrouping though—no one is! I'm ashamed of it now, but I would do thoughtlessly cruel things back then, like making gay jokes. I didn't understand how pointing out people's differences and repeating harmful stereotypes for a cheap laugh is dehumanizing and can even put people in danger.

I didn't hate anyone, but there were definitely groups of people I just didn't understand or feel I could relate to. As an athlete, for example, I wanted to be strong (even when I wasn't healthy).

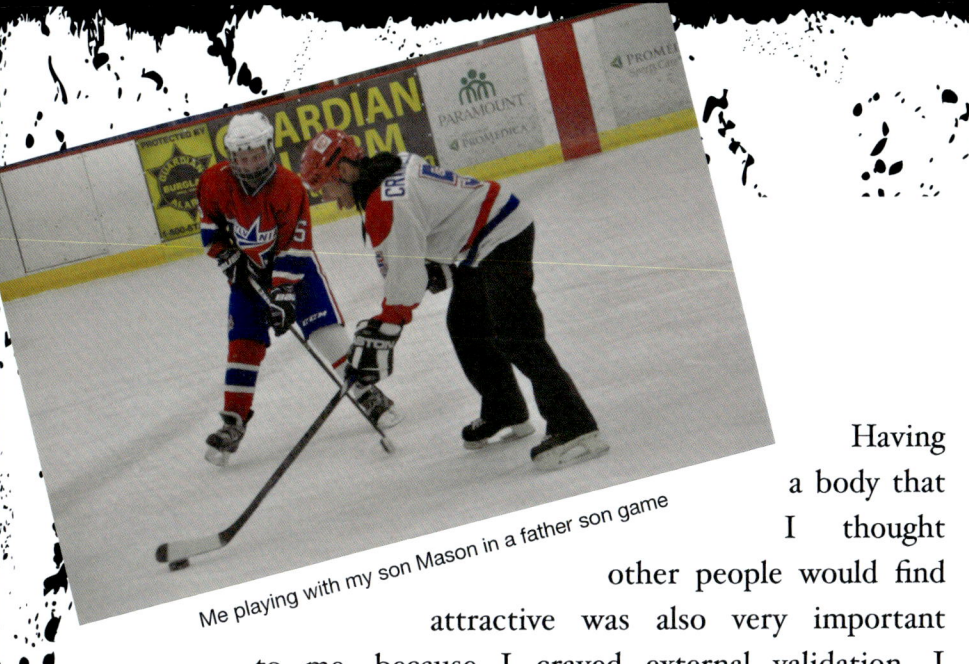
Me playing with my son Mason in a father son game

Having a body that I thought other people would find attractive was also very important to me, because I craved external validation. I couldn't understand how people could possibly develop weight problems—the idea of not working out or overeating was totally alien to me. After all, I kept going to the gym, even when I was so messed up on drugs and alcohol that my body was falling apart.

In my sobriety, my compassion and ability to empathize shot through the roof. I started to understand that none of us were that different—that we were all just struggling, and we used different coping mechanisms to try and deal with the pain we felt. As a counselor, I could see everyone's humanity shine through whatever else they were dealing with. I'd been hurting, so I'd used cocaine; he'd been hurting, so he'd used food. I'd felt abandoned by my mom's suicide; she'd felt abandoned by her parents' reaction when she came out of the closet. Sure, I'd never been morbidly obese or a lesbian, but those differences were superficial. We could connect on a deeper level than the labels, and my labels didn't make me any more or less than them.

Choosing to heal from trauma is about practicing empathy. By understanding that we are all connected because we have all experienced pain, you flip trauma on its head. Masking your pain with drugs and alcohol kept you locked inside yourself and alienated; developing empathy gives it a purpose and helps you understand yourself and other people on new levels. When you build your compassion, you make the world a kinder, better place, and your own world becomes much richer and comprehensive.

People can't be bad any more than they can be weak, because we can always start making good choices. We can also make bad choices (people in pain often do), and we can hurt other people terribly. We make mistakes, but it is essential that we don't become our mistakes.

I was a nice kid. I was a very giving kid. I was a kindhearted kid. I was an intelligent kid...but I was a broken kid. I had tremendous anger issues. I was physically violent. When I started using drugs, I'd be fun for the first couple of beers, and then absolute rage would come out...then this crazy, manic energy, then suicidal depression. Same cycle, all the time. It was like a tornado that just wreaked havoc on anybody who was in my life. The emotional devastation I caused a lot of innocent people is just catastrophic.

I did those things. I made those choices. I will never stop being sorry for that, but if I let myself be paralyzed by shame, I could not have gotten help. I would not have made better choices. I would not be able to help others today.

Balancing our low self-esteem with taking responsibility for our actions is complicated. We can talk about what we've done and what to do and that is different than who we are. Accept your responsibility, take appropriate actions, and make strong choices moving forward. Keep moving forward. Keep making yourself and the world around you better. Keep building your value. Stay positive and don't let shame paralyze you. Shame can prevent you from taking the necessary steps to get help. Disruptive behaviors are a direct display of emotional turmoil that needs to be addressed. Having the courage to address emotional hurt is an example of self-care that can lead to not only sobriety, but productivity throughout life.

**YOU ARE NOT A BAD PERSON. CHOOSING TO BELIEVE YOU ARE A BAD PERSON WILL ONLY LEAD YOU TO MAKE MORE BAD CHOICES, TO HURT MORE PEOPLE. CHOOSE TO HEAL, TO MAKE BETTER CHOICES, TO MAKE THE WORLD A BETTER PLACE.**

## HOW CAN I DEAL WITH GRIEF?

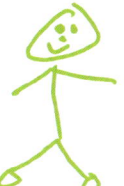

"You're not going to die in my garage. You got to leave."

I'd been up and on a bender for a couple days at this point, and Kevin's words stung my pride. I look back now and think, good for him—it takes guts to tell your friends that you don't want to stand by and watch them kill themselves.

Kevin was probably six or seven years younger than me, but we got to know each other through hockey. He was a big pot smoker, and we'd drink together in his parent's garage, which had been converted into a nice living space.

He was with me on April 12, 1993. We were heading to see Guns 'N Roses. At the bend in the road on 75 North in Monroe, Michigan, right before it goes under a bridge, he offered me a pill from his handful, warning me to take just one. I threw them all back and we went to see Guns 'N Roses. Well, he went to go see Guns 'N Roses; that curve in the road was the last thing I remembered. He found me out in the parking lot after everybody was gone, blacked out and leaning up against a streetlight. I remember him telling me, "God, we were so mad, we were gonna leave you there. We were sick and tired of you doing this crap to us." They didn't. The next morning, I got arrested on my third DUI and finally chose sobriety.

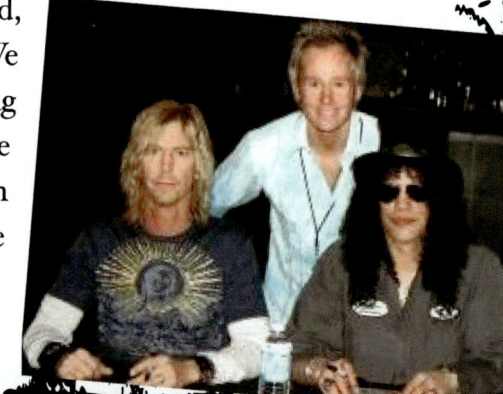

Me with Slash and Duff from Guns and Roses years later

(Years later, I sat in Duff McKagan's dressing room and told him about this night, about how I saw him play but didn't remember it. He laughed and told me he didn't remember it either, and it hit me straight in the gut. It reminded me that, despite all the glitz, I was sitting here with another man who had struggled through a painful addiction. We were both able to be in that room because we'd chosen not to do drugs or drink any longer.)

Kevin and I spent a lot of time working out together and playing hockey after that, but it was like our lives started to switch: I was getting sober, and he started getting into opiates.

He came into Racing for Recovery probably ten or twelve years ago with some legal issues. He had to clean up, but as soon as he took care of the courts, he never came back. I think I only saw him once after that, briefly. We were linked for life through the friendship we'd built, and he knew I'd always be there for him, that the doors at Racing for Recovery would always be open to him. We just had nothing in common anymore.

On a recent Sunday, I was at a professional dinner when I got a text. One of our friends found Kevin's body.

My phone started blowing up with texts and calls after that—other friends reaching out, asking if I'd heard, what I'd heard, what details I had. I was sad and angry, and I quickly became frustrated.

What happened? He never chose sobriety, and the consequence was his life.

The details of his final moments just didn't matter. He didn't get to die of old age, surrounded by his loved ones. He didn't die happy. He died with drugs still in his brain, and now his son, whose got my old high school goalie position, has to live with a father-shaped hole in his heart.

On Tuesday, I got a call from Jason—he was out of jail, and this time, he was going to do it. It was a follow-up to the letter he'd sent me a few weeks back, and it was just the news I needed. Jason had once celebrated sixth months of sobriety waiting for me at the finish line of a half-IRONMAN. I'd given him my medal—a placeholder until he could win his own. He was important to me and the Racing for Recovery community.

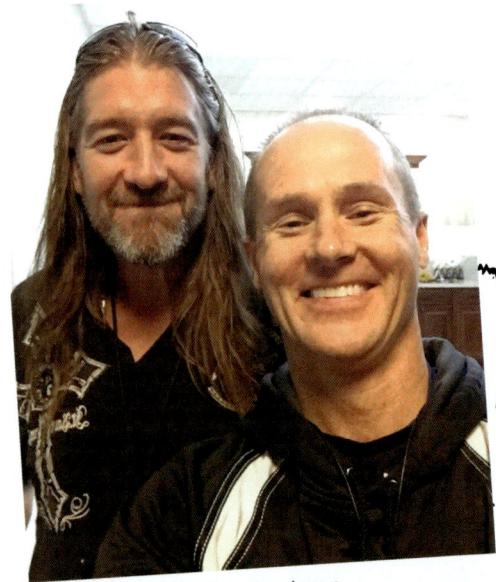

Less than twenty-four hours later, Jason overdosed and died.

This wasn't how Jason's story should have ended. It's not how Kevin's story should have

I miss you Jason.

3/1/19

Todd

I'll be out of jail on the 12th of March, and I'll have 65 days clean and be on the Vivitrol shot.

I want, ~~~~ no I need to be back envolved with Racing for Recovery.

I know you heard from Joes. He's getting out before me

I'm ready to recommit myself to Sustainable Sobriety and your program.

I don't have another recovery in me. This has to be the one that lasts a life time.

I don't know what I have to do to get in the Hotel, Just tell me when I get out and I'll do it. I cant be on the East side any more. Not right now.

So please let me help myself talk to you soon.

JASON Oook

ended. They had both reached out for help, they'd both made some amazing choices. But they both made the wrong choice last week, and they paid the ultimate price. These weren't "bad guys." They were great guys. They weren't weak. I had been proud to stand beside both of them, and I wish—so much—that I still had the chance to stand next to either of them today.

Choosing drugs and alcohol kills people. That's a fact that we face every day at Racing for Recovery. The collateral damage of these choices, the grief and trauma of family and friends, is immense. We know no one could have chosen sobriety for Kevin and Jason except Kevin and Jason, but it still hurts. How do you deal with that type of grief?

Choosing to heal and help others heal from grief requires a lot of listening, empathy, and support. You can also make this pain meaningful and honor the ones you have lost by taking whatever is salvageable and using it to help somebody else. Share your story. Show people what the consequences of their wrong choices could be. Help them understand. Pain pulls us inward, and makes everything else seem far away, and hurt people often cannot see beyond themselves. When your grief is strong enough to tear you apart, that is power. I have seen what happens when you harness it.

A member of the Racing for Recovery community, a woman named Karena, recently called me right after she found her daughter's body. Terah, her daughter, my client, had been in the Racing for Recovery community for years, but she'd stopped. I invited the mother to come to our support group when she was ready.

I was surprised but glad when she showed up just two days later. She'd brought her other two daughters with her. Their pain was raw and intense and obvious. I hoped that we would be able to help, comfort, and guide them.

Shortly after the meeting started, Karena stood up.

"Look at my face," she said.

Everyone in the room searched her face. I admit, it was hard. She was in so much pain that even engaging with it hurt.

"Look at my daughters' faces."

The daughters were still sitting, so I caught sight of other people in the crowd as we glanced towards them. Many of us looked grief-stricken, even those who had never met the dead woman. It was impossible not to empathize with her family's pain, to imagine our own if we lost one of the people we loved most.

"And remember this if you ever think of using drugs again."

This woman was grieving intensely—literally, physically weakened and sick from a wound to her soul that was still gaping open.

She'd had no time to adjust to her new normal, a world without her child. She had not even buried her daughter yet. No one on this planet would have faulted her for staying in bed for a month, and she didn't owe anyone in that room anything.

But, in a true act of selflessness and grace, she made her pain into a powerful and incredible gift. She used it to heal other people. She created beauty and hope and power out of something unspeakably tragic and ugly. She made us understand, on an atomic level, something that can never be fully expressed in words. She made us better people. Though we will never know who or how many, I know Karena saved lives that day.

## ...DO I NEED TO BE AN IRON MAN? CAN I? SHOULD I?!?!

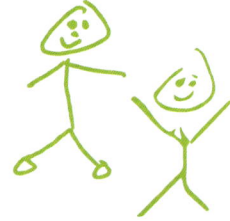

As I sat on the flight to Denver, Colorado, on June 6, 2018, with my daughter Skylar, I was overcome with gratitude. We were flying with her best friend Allie (my fifth child) and a Racing for Recovery crew: Stephen, Jeff and Rachel. If you would have told me years ago, when I was living in my car, that I would be doing this today, I would have told you that you were insane!

I never thought I was going to be alive, let alone have a loving family and a successful recovery program.

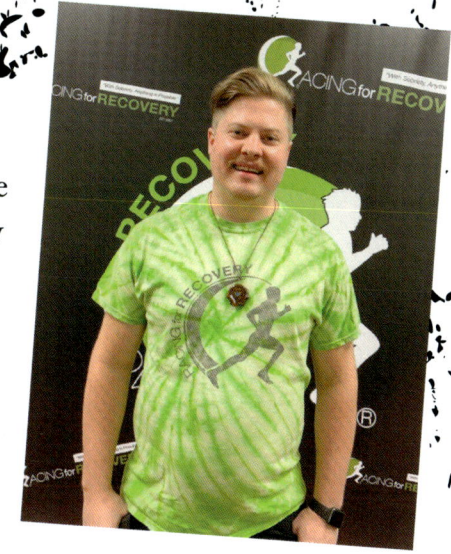

Stephen sat across the aisle from me. As I gazed over at him, I couldn't help but recall the desperate state he and his family were in just three years ago. It is inspiring to witness his work through addiction and with Racing for Recovery. He now helps others who are in his former shoes. His sense of humor and compassion for himself and others is awesome to be around.

When we arrived in Denver, seven additional members picked us up and took us to where we were staying in Boulder. I checked my phone: My stepmom left me a kind voicemail, which brought tears to my eyes. Our relationship is an example of true healing, and it feels awesome. There is no hurt, no anger, no resentment, nothing negative between us. Although it wasn't always the case, now there is only kindness, love, peace and happiness. Time and sobriety heal wounds and lead us to places we often find unimaginable. Mom actually started me on the IRONMAN path, many, many years ago. I played hockey, and I got one trophy a year. When Mom took up running, she started getting trophies every week, and I definitely wanted a piece of that action.

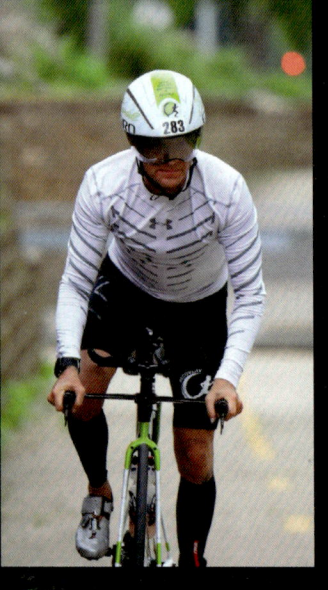

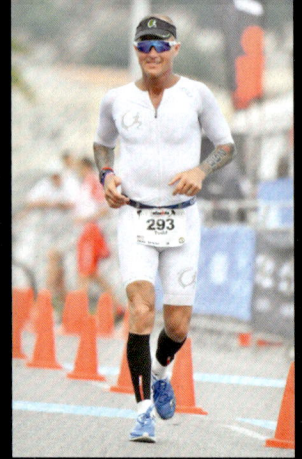

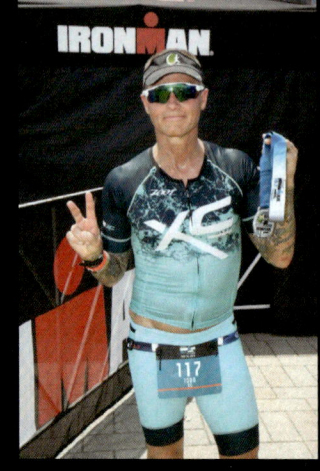

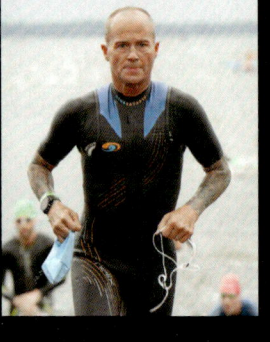

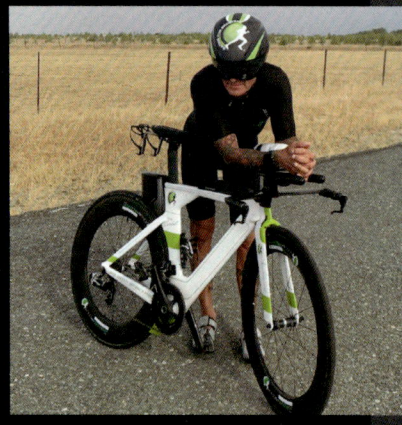

Clockwise from top left: Promoting Racing for Recovery through IRONMAN events in Wisconsin, France, Tennessee, and filming in Spain

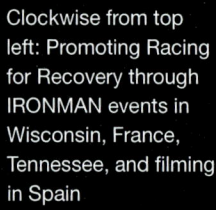

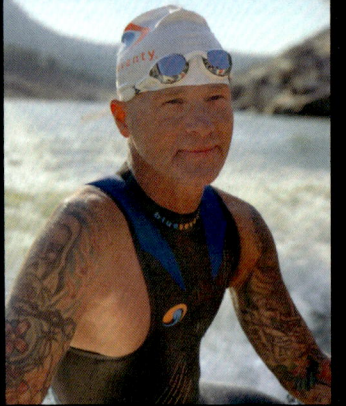

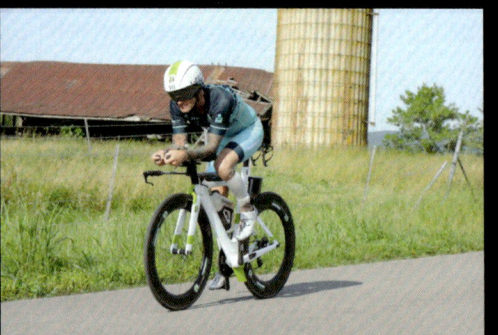

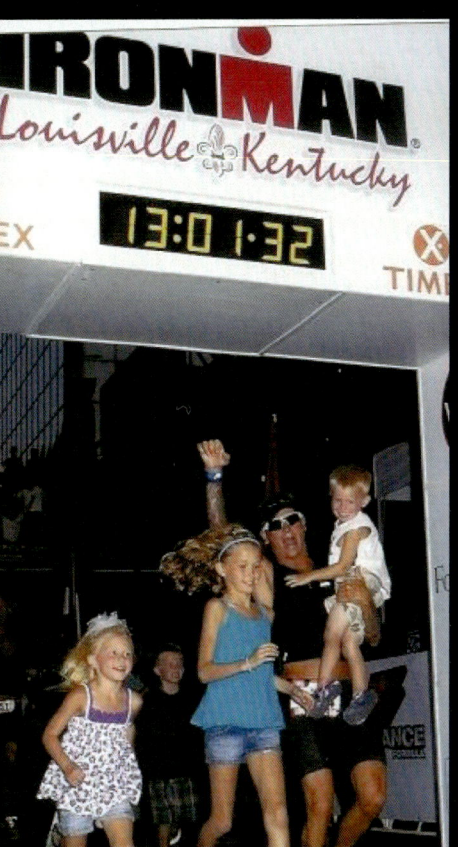

13:01:32

IRONMAN
Louisville Kentucky

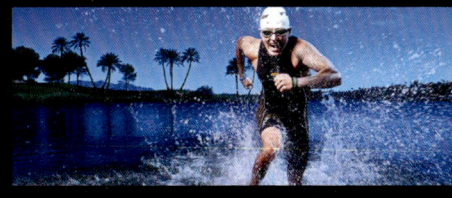

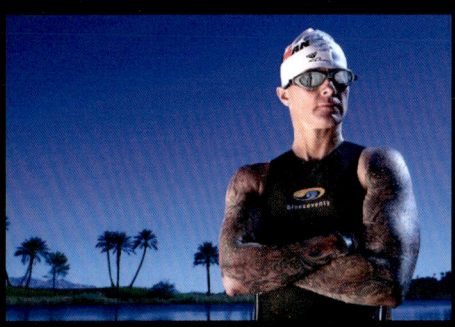

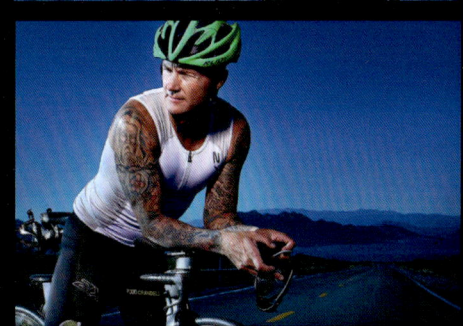

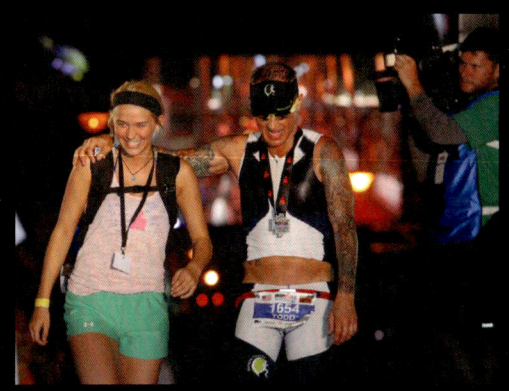

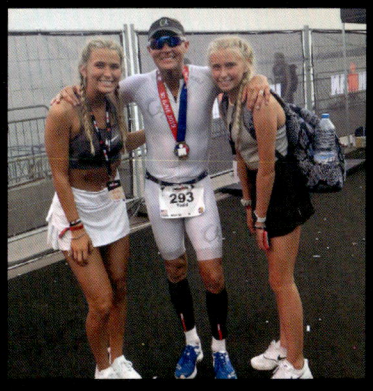

Finishing IRONMAN Louisville, Kentucky, Melbourne, Australia and Nice, France.

This brings me to the IRONMAN itself. I have been doing these crazy things since 1999 and each one has had a purpose, personal and/or professional. I am now sponsored by Mercy Health, which, like Racing for Recovery, provides service to those in need. I am proud to represent them as I compete in events around the world, and their sponsorship has been critical.

I have been through emotionally difficult times while competing in IRONMAN triathlons; my spirit has been broken, my marriage has struggled, and my body has been beaten-up. In the past, I would endure these events because I felt a sense of duty. I was obligated to all of those involved. Trudging through, however, came with a price. This time, however, I felt gratitude. I am blessed to have come to IRONMAN Boulder with a healthy body, an amazing marriage, and with success stories from Racing for Recovery.

I am so grateful that my work and sponsorship from Mercy Medical allowed me to do this and bring my support crew of ten members and two coworkers. During the race, I am dependent on my team instead of being the one who provides the support. It is satisfying to experience that role reversal, and it only deepens my appreciation for these incredible people.

I was glad that they were able to enjoy their trip to Boulder. They went skydiving, whitewater rafting, hiking, sightseeing. The trip really was a pretty perfect example of the full life we can live when we're sober. This is one of the main points I do my best to convey to others: Sobriety is not just about not using drugs. It is about living in sobriety and doing things you never thought you would do.

Now I feel proud, grateful, relieved, excited, and overall just peaceful. Yes, I still jump from Oh my God, can I do this? to I can and will do this! These mental challenges are normal for such extreme endurance events, and they have helped me transfer this dedication to my work. I've learned to dig deep within and go to a place that requires mental and emotional toughness. The reward is an unbelievable sense of accomplishment when I cross the finish line. Despite being in pain from head to toe, when the race is done, I rejoice.

I still enjoy the personal achievements, but it is the impact on people that motivates me. As I prepared mentally for IRONMAN Boulder, I reflected on a recent event at IRONMAN Chattanooga 70.3. I met a girl and fellow plant-based triathlete who said, "Your first book saved my life and I am here because of your story and the mission of Racing for Recovery." **THAT IS WHY I DO THESE RACES!** This is the point, the impact on real people. One bonus to the Boulder IRONMAN was the media coverage. Our success stories were featured on NBC and FOX News Denver.

I've only ever failed to finish one IRONMAN race—the one

in Malaysia the day before my youngest daughter was born. I almost quit IRONMAN Chattanooga in 2016, and it would have been one of the worst choices I've made in sobriety.

I hadn't been training for the race the way I needed to because I'd been embracing the opportunities on the business side, but I'd promised a client we'd do it together. I got in the water for the swim knowing I was unprepared, and on the very first stroke, I lost my wedding ring. I got out of the water and found out my client had quit before he'd even finished the swim—I was on my own. I was hurting bad by the first lap of the marathon and I was ready to quit, and Melissa told me to get out there and finish. I got fed up in the next lap, and I sat in the SAG van for a minute and started justifying all the reasons I didn't need to finish—and then I got out and finished, because I knew I did need to. My family was there, waiting at the finish line, even though it took me so long to meet up with them that Mason looked at Melissa and asked "Mom, why does Dad have to suck so bad?" Later that night, after I fell on my face in exhaustion, he told me it was time to retire.

That whole race was like one giant metaphor for the hardest days of sobriety. Even if it starts out rocky, you gotta keep going. Even if your buddy drops out, you gotta keep going. Even if you're tired and falling all over yourself, you've gotta keep going. Even if your support system is fed up with you, you gotta keep going. You've got to make the right choice, even when you've fully justified the wrong choice in your head. Sobriety is awesome, but the rewards you're going to pull in are so much bigger than you can imagine. Finishing that tough race was great, but do you know my real reward? *I GOT TO BUILD MY DREAM.*

See, we'd just toured the building that would become the Racing for Recovery center, and A.J., a counselor I'd been working with, one of the most instrumental people in the organization since the moment we opened our doors, was ready to hand in his resignation and devote himself to building up Racing for Recovery into what it is today. Without him, I wouldn't have even been able to consider moving into the building and giving it my all. We knew each other professionally, but we were getting ready to take a massive leap of faith together. A.J. told me later that he never would have quit his job and teamed up with me if I'd quit that race. He never would have been able to trust me to work through the hard times. Words are great, but actions are everything; if I'd let myself down at the race that day, I would have let down the thousands of people who've been able to find help, resources, and sobriety in this building.

After finishing IRONMAN Boulder, joy filled my heart and my mind was overcome with gratitude. I finished the event at high altitude in extreme heat. My body was spent but my spirits were high.

Boulder was the worst of my 29 IRONMAN finishes. My time, 16 hours 20 minutes, was close to the 17-hour limit. I don't care about time, I just wanted my finish to be official, and logging another official finish was amazing. Most important, however, was the experience I had with my team and peers. Hearing the cheers of support was amazing and kept me going through this particularly arduous race.

By end of 2019, I'll have finished thirty-one IRONMAN races and fifty IRONMAN 70.3 races. My fiftieth 70.3 will be at the World Championships in Nice, France, and my thirty-first full-length IRONMAN will be at the World Championships in Kona—the two biggest events in triathlon, within four weeks of each other. (Of course, I will be taking members of Racing for Recovery to both!) The challenge isn't merely the events themselves, which are demanding. They tax me physically, mentally, emotionally, and take up time and resources. More significant is the time required to train for the events. At my age (over fifty), and with the time demands of running Racing for Recovery, it is challenging to put in the necessary hours to train for each event. These are grueling races and demand that competitors do more than roll out of bed and show up at the starting line. My focus today is sobriety and expanding sobriety to those who need our help.

I fully enjoy watching the friendships that are made in sobriety. People often come in feeling broken and defeated. After time with recovery, they regain their families, return to school, gain and retain employment, and make better friends than they've ever had. Some even venture into ambitious endeavors like, running marathons and competing in triathlons. These people become inspirations for others and improve the overall human experience relating to substance abuse. When people are inspired in their lives, they have the highest success rates. Self-destruction doesn't even register at that point.

Exercise and caring for your body are so important to me, to how I understand my own sobriety and life. I've seen it be and become as important to many other people too. I certainly don't think you need to be a triathlete to be sober. (But if that's your dream, you should definitely go for it!) But I know that exercise it a critical part of living a balanced, healthy, holistic life in sobriety, for both the well-known physical aspects and the healing mental connections.

When I chose to use drugs and alcohol, I punished, disrespected, and abandoned my body. I set a goal to self-destruct too many times to count. I literally poisoned myself, day after day, for thirteen years. I thought I wanted to die, and I consciously and subconsciously pushed my body towards that edge. It stubbornly held in there; it kept me tethered to this world; it waited for me to come around and decide to get my heart and my mind in the game. It kept me alive, even when I refused to give it much to go on, even when I was directly sabotaging its efforts.

As an endurance athlete, I've honored the strength and worth my body showed me I had long before I believed or appreciated it. I respect that it is capable of more than I think possible. I try to push it beyond its limits, and it shows me over and over where my self-limiting beliefs are. It teaches me about the connection between my willpower, my mind, and my muscles. Exercising my body is physical, yes, but it is also emotional and spiritual and communal. It's truly holistic.

**RECONNECTING (OR CONNECTING FOR THE VERY FIRST TIME) WITH YOUR BODY IS A CRUCIAL ELEMENT TO CHOOSING SOBRIETY AND CHOOSING TO HEAL.** Whatever external trauma you experienced and internalized that led you to choose to drink and do drugs, you took your body hostage. It showed up for you every day, even when you did not choose to show up for yourself. You forgot, or never realized in the first place, how powerful your body is, all the incredible things that you are capable of doing with it. Finding that power through exercise is a step that both stands alone and will propel you through every other choice you need to make.

## HOW DO I HEAL WITHOUT GETTING SICK?

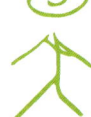

I was still shaking the water out of my ears from an early morning two-mile swim when my first client of the day walked into my office.

"I feel awful. Like, physically. This is the worst I've ever felt," she said, settling her energy drink beside her chair.

My client is new—but not brand new. She's chosen sobriety, and she's choosing to heal, and, like many before, she's figuring out that it can be pretty exhausting.

"Tell me about your breakfast," I said, throwing my own banana peel into the trash.

Being a counselor is a little like being a detective. I like to ask the questions, even when I can deduce the answers from the evidence: Her coat smelled like the cigarette she'd disposed of on her way in the door, and there was a tell-tale spot of a donut's powdered sugar on the lapel.

People in recovery often talk about withdrawal from drugs and alcohol. That makes sense; a lot of us relied on the drugs we were consuming to power us through the day. Drugs do a crappy job with keeping us healthy, but without those drugs, your body might not know where to go for energy and regulation. That was my main driver to start running when I chose sobriety—I felt awful. I was committed, but I was sick—literally, physically sick. I needed my body to be able to keep up with the life I knew I wanted to live in sobriety. Sitting in low energy, smoky rooms with stale coffee and donuts wasn't going to make me feel physically better. I needed to train my body to run off something besides anger and sadness and drugs.

Choosing to heal can be a surprise double-whammy for your body. We talked about how your brain experiences trauma as real, physical hurt, and being physically hurt takes a lot out of you; anxiety and depression are natural (though not really helpful) responses to pain. If you want to heal, you have to face the trauma and see it for everything it is—nothing to mask it, no bandages. If it feels at first like you're walking around with an open wound—well, that's because, in some ways, you are.

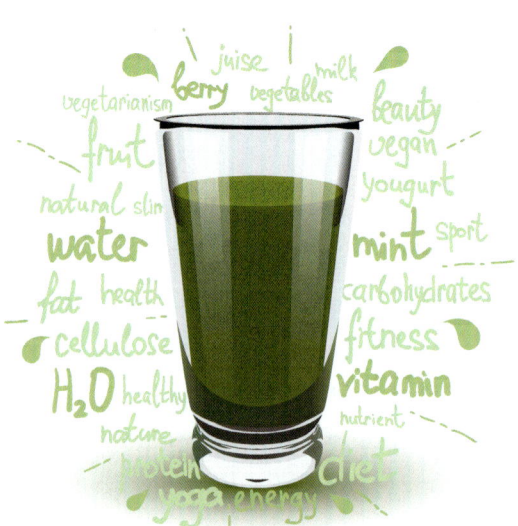

Healing is an emotional process, but it's also a physical process. When you're committed to looking inside yourself, it is crucial to build and maintain your health through your lifestyle. You can't expect to think clearly and heal emotionally if you're putting junk in your body—it just doesn't work. If you are living right, exercising, taking vitamins, and eating right, you're fueling your body for healing. You're less likely to be anxious and depressed, and when you do go through tough emotional moments, you're better able to return quickly to a good place inside your head that you can continue healing from.

I'm a licensed, certified IRONMAN coach, so I can put together pretty great plans for people with respect to swimming, biking, and running. Everyone's dietary needs are individualized, though, so we don't pass out food plans at Racing for Recovery. We have resources and movies for people to explore when they're ready.

The nutritional education I have is based on my own hard-earned experience, learning my body as an endurance athlete. I've been fine-tuning now for twenty-six years, and it's still cool to think about and put in action each day. I know how I'm going to feel at every point based on what I'm doing, what the differences are in my mood and energy level based on if I swam or ran, what time my energy is the highest and what time it starts to diminish. It's based off food and exercise, sure, but it's also grounded and balanced with every other choice I make throughout the day—spiritual, family, communal. I've gotten to know my body and what it needs—when it wants Niacin and Vitamin C and D, when and how much water I need to take in, when a banana is just what the internal doctor ordered. I am continuously improving my health and wellness and diet, and I have my own IRONMAN coaches that help me with very specific, detailed training plans for that type of regimen.

IRONMAN triathletes are committed to our sport. We spend a lot of time and resources finding the most aerodynamic helmets and wetsuits with the least drag, structuring our workouts to maximize the benefits and performance and hiring the best coaches. We wake up early, time our splits, measure our heart rates, and tune our bikes—and that's before we even travel, all over the world, to the events.

But what goes into our bodies? What we eat affects not only how we perform on race day, but how we feel 365 days a year and our overall health. The focus on in-race nutrition has grown in recent years. (I know I've been interviewed by more than one curious reporter about how I'm fueling myself through race day!)

I'm one of a growing number of IRONMEN committed to a vegan, plant-based diet, whether I'm pushing myself through Kona or relaxing at home in Ohio.

I still run into some people who are genuinely confused by the idea of a vegan athlete, who believe that I must be sacrificing some major health benefits for some other purpose. I can empathize with that—I used to think so too.

In sobriety, I live my life with empathy, humility, and compassion.

Even on the darkest days of my addiction, though, when I couldn't really appreciate humanity, I've always felt compassionate towards animals. The way that compassion was at odds with diet made me uneasy for years, but I was an athlete. I'd grown up at the hockey rink. The ideas that building and maintaining muscle requires proteins, and that proteins were synonymous with slabs of animal muscle, were deeply ingrained.

As an endurance athlete who has been vegan for three years, I can tell you that **I WAS WRONG.** I feel better now than when I ate meat. I perform better, I recover more quickly, and I enjoy racing more. I've seen changes in myself, my body, and my abilities that blow my mind.

I had already done a lot of research and made adjustments to my diet by the day I went vegan (February 1, 2016—the second most important date in my healing journey, only surpassed by the day I chose sobriety). I was still surprised to find how drastically my plant-based diet improved my athletic performance. My results weren't a fluke, either. I've

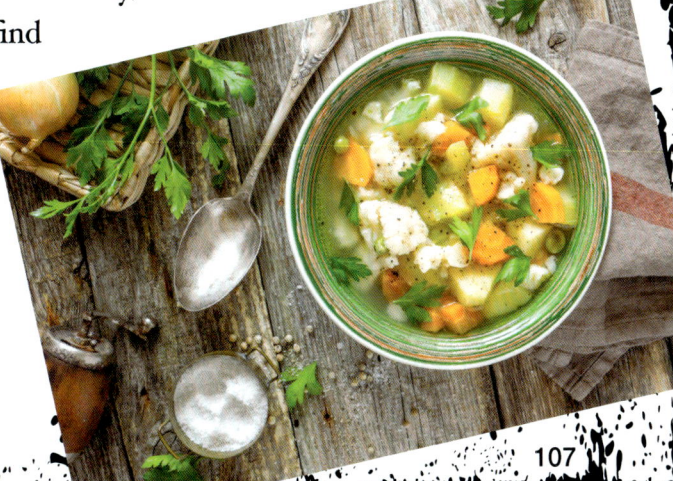

seen the same changes in other people at Racing for Recovery, and studies have now shown that a vegan diet improves performance among endurance athletes. We can set new personal records while being healthier, feeling and looking better, and doing more for the world around us.

The physical improvements that a vegan diet provides benefit nearly everyone, endurance athlete or not. Even with no increase in activity or change in body weight, vegan diets reduce body fat and create leaner body mass, increasing our aerobic capacity and the amount of oxygen in our bloodstreams, making all motions easier.

The human body stores energy as glycogen, a carbohydrate, then uses it to fuel our performances. As anyone who has ever 'hit the wall' can attest, running out of carbohydrate stores can quickly end a race day. Plant-based diets are rich in complex carbohydrates, beefing up our glycogen stores, providing us more energy and decreasing fatigue. They lower blood viscosity and increase arterial elasticity and diameter. That allows more blood to flow to and from our muscles, making it easier to deliver all this extra oxygen and plant-based carbohydrate stores where it needs to go.

From massages to foam rollers to cryotherapy to compression boots and socks, post-race recovery is a big part of endurance athletics, and vegan diets don't let us down. When we exert our muscles, they produce 'free radicals,' molecules that can damage our DNA, lead to atherosclerosis, cause fatigue, and otherwise impair recovery. A vegan diet contains more antioxidants, which help neutralize the effects of those free radicals. As strange as it may sound, eating more blueberries might help your race more than new shoes or a new bike. Vegan diets also improve recovery by reducing the inflammation in our bodies caused by exercise.

Plant-based diets reduce lipid concentrations in our blood (cholesterol), reduce blood pressure, and improve blood glucose control. Not to be dramatic, but adopting a plant-based diet can save a runner's life. It helps reverse atherosclerosis (fatty deposits that narrow coronary arteries). Endurance athletes actually have more advanced atherosclerosis and heart damage than sedentary people, and these problems worsen with age. Despite very regularly exercising our hearts, we actually have an increased risk of heart attack. The alternative—high cholesterol, hypertension, increased body-mass index (BMI), type 2 diabetes, and clogged arteries—generally makes for shorter, less healthy, and less pleasant lives.

Meat and dairy are simply not good for us or the planet. Consumption of red meat and processed meats significantly increases the risk of colorectal cancer, which kills more than 50,000 people per year in the United States alone. Eating red meat just once a week increases the risk of colorectal cancer by nearly forty percent. Grilling or pan-frying meats further increases cancer risks. Nearly forty percent of Americans are obese, defined as having a BMI as 30 or higher. White meat, long thought to be healthier than red meat, has an equally negative impact on cholesterol, according to recent studies. Overfishing has cut fish populations nearly in half since 1970, threatening both the sustainability of fishing and all marine life, and those that are left are filled with the elevated levels of mercury, polychlorinated biphenyls (PCBs), heavy metals, and microplastics that pollute our waters. The high concentration of saturated fats in dairy products increases the risk of prostate cancer and heart disease. For the growing population of people with lactose intolerance, dairy consumption is also associated with increased risk of lung cancer, breast cancer, and ovarian cancer. The standard American diet (SAD) leads to a short, unhealthy, unpleasant life. Though nearly all endurance athletes eat a healthier diet than the SAD, veganism offers the best alternative for all of us, athlete, non-athlete, and non-human alike.

Plant-based diets, rich in complex carbohydrates and low in saturated fats, improve digestion, help us feel fuller after eating, and improve sleep, which positively affects immune function, metabolism, memory, learning, and more.

Eating a plant-based diet is easy and accessible, and veganism isn't confined to a very small subset of the population anymore. From nutritional guides to plant-based recipes, resources for people looking to make the switch are everywhere. We all dig into grains, vegetables, fruits, nuts, and beans—no changes needed there. From the grocery store to your favorite restaurant, meat alternatives and vegan options are more widely available than ever. Even fast food chains centered around meat, like McDonald's and Burger King, are increasing their non-meat offerings. Whenever I hop in the van and head out of town for a Racing for Recovery event, one of the first things I ask Siri to investigate is the nearest Chipotle. I ate a vegan bowl from Chipotle every single day I was at IRONMAN Atlantic City. Eating fast food every day isn't ideal, but the widespread availability of vegan substitutes everywhere just makes it easier to maintain this diet, wherever you go.

Talking about and advocating for a vegan diet is a trickier thing than it should be. I don't force veganism on anyone. I believe in helping people by continuously offering my experiences, just like I did with drugs and alcohol. Taking care of your body with both exercise and nutrition is an important part of a balanced, healthy, sober, holistic lifestyle, but making it vegan is my suggestion, not a position of the Racing for Recovery program. As people see the awesome results I'm getting as an endurance athlete and as a person with this diet, they make some of the same choices in their own lives. Training for an IRONMAN—or any race—isn't an official part of the Racing for Recovery program either, but they are a big part of my journey, and I talk about them freely and openly. At the end of the day, choosing what your own ideal holistic lifestyle looks like is the key to your sobriety.

I have had incredible success with my plant-based diet for health and athletic purposes, but I also strongly believe that it is the right choice to make for environmental and compassionate reasons. These positions can make some people feel upset or uncomfortable, which is not my purpose, but not sharing them would be completely against the spirit of everything I've built— it would be dishonest. It would be hiding things that I know are true for the comfort of people who want to make easier decisions that I believe hurt them and hurt the world around them.

It takes 660 gallons of water to make one cheeseburger. Thirty-thousand miles of river in the U.S. are polluted beyond repair with pig and cow manure. Meat and dairy provide only 18% of global calories and 37% of protein, but occupy 83% of the world's farmland and account for 60% of agriculture's greenhouse gas emissions. Eating meat not only significantly contributes to climate change—it is killing the world around us, plant and animal alike. Biking through Nice, filming a documentary in Madrid, even scurrying out of the Vegas sun to meet Aerosmith, I'm overwhelmed with gratitude for how beautiful our planet is and how amazing life can be. Doing my part to keep it all going with every forkful that hits my mouth feels like the very least I owe us all.

In order to support our demand for cheap meat, animals are kept in miserable, torturous conditions, stacked on top of one another, often unable to even turn around. The filthy conditions would be lethal to any creature, so they are pumped with antibiotics to prevent widespread livestock death, generating an incredible amount of toxic pollutant waste. The methane released creates germs resistant to antibiotics, contaminates soil and drinking water, and contributes to climate change. The conditions in factory farms are so repulsive that very few people with other options will agree to work there. Many of the workers are exploited undocumented immigrants, who are often subjected to cruel treatment by unscrupulous employers. These farmworkers, some of whom are much younger than my own children, risk infection, injury, and death from the animals and their waste. These factories chew through innocent vulnerability, human and animal alike.

Statistics do not adequately capture the nearly incomprehensible scale and pervasive cruelty of American industrial agriculture as they slaughter billions of animals for human consumption each year. Broiler chickens, the animal most commonly killed, grow to maturity in barely five weeks. They often spend their entire lives in areas no bigger than a piece of paper. They cannot support the weight of their selectively bred breasts and wings. They have their beaks cut off to prevent them from pecking themselves or each other to death as they go insane from the sounds of suffering and conditions that surround them. Their deaths may include being boiled alive. Hens bred to lay eggs endure similar conditions, just for longer than their broiler cousins. Cows and pigs, who are remarkably intelligent but exempted from most animal cruelty laws, are sometimes kicked, slapped, punched, and beaten. Pigs, who share many behaviors and intellectual abilities with dogs and chimpanzees, are killed by the hundreds of millions each year after being kept in miserable conditions. Cows, who have the ability to reason and exhibit anxiety when kept in isolation, have metal bolts driven through their skulls before they're raised to the ceiling by the chains attached to their hind legs and their throats are slit to drain any remaining blood.

I'm not sharing this information to make you feel bad about yourself or your personal choice and history. I'm sharing it because I think you're awesome, and I know that you're reading this book because you want to live the best life possible. I think about other horror shows that have happened throughout history, like slavery and the Holocaust. If I'd been alive and contributing to that type of pain and suffering, I would have wanted someone to tell me about it honestly and explain how I could stop and fight to end it. I think our kids and their kids are going to look back at this time in history and be really sad and angry that this happened right under our noses, and that not enough people stood up nearly quickly enough to say 'no.' Choosing healing is about making decisions for yourself that will help you balance your life and make the world a better place.

When I became vegan, it enhanced every principle I live for in sobriety. It gave me more compassion than I'd ever thought was possible—compassion for innocent beings that don't want to die, that don't deserve to die, that are being tortured and murdered by the millions every day so that we can poison ourselves and the environment. I became vegan for my health, for the animals, and because I want to save our planet. I truly believe that when people understand the benefits of doing this without judgment or fear, our world will be a better place. It's made me a better person, a better husband, father, athlete, and counselor.

And it's made me a much better friend to my third son, Milo.

Milo came into our lives two years

ago, after I flippantly agreed to let my daughter get a pet potbellied pig—hypothetically, if she ever happened to stumble across one that really needed a home. She pretty quickly "stumbled across" one, and we bonded immediately. He's brilliant. He does tricks, he rings a bell when he needs to go outside. He's part of the family—he even has his own room. He's brought so much into my life, including a very real sense of the intelligence, warmth, and personality that animals—even ones considered "livestock"—have.

When I sat down on February 1, 2016, and started watching documentaries and paying more attention to the meat and dairy industry than I'd ever allowed myself, I hadn't had a steak in twenty years. By the end of the day, I knew I was finished consuming animals for good.

Refusing to take part any longer in a system I could not defend was clearly the compassionate, ethical, and environmentally-friendly option. The health and athletic benefits of following my heart and my conscious make this a choice I feel I can fully endorse and recommend that you consider.

Addiction consumes your life and robs your body of nourishment. Choosing to heal means making choices to nourish your brain and your body and your spirit. Whatever decisions that you make about feeding yourself, remember that this is the fuel you'll be using to build the life you want and accomplish awesome things.

If you take care of your body, every other choice that you make will be easier and more joyful.

## WHAT IF I JUST WANT TO DIE?

**IF YOU ARE IN CRISIS, CALL THE TOLL-FREE NATIONAL SUICIDE PREVENTION LIFELINE (NSPL) AT 1-800-273-TALK (8255), AVAILABLE TWENTY-FOUR HOURS A DAY, SEVEN DAYS A WEEK. THE SERVICE IS AVAILABLE TO ANYONE. ALL CALLS ARE CONFIDENTIAL.**

The day my daughter Madison was born, I flew home from an IRONMAN in Malaysia that I didn't finish and shouldn't have even gone to in the first place. I made it to the hospital less than two hours before she was born.

I left my beautiful house and my amazing family early in the morning on my daughter's sixteenth birthday. I drove to the Racing for Recovery building, my literal dream-come-true, and hit the pool for a morning swim surrounded by awesome sober friends.

And I was overcome by suicidal thoughts, pummeling myself about a choice I wish I'd made differently sixteen years ago that could have (but didn't) resulted in a crappy consequence.

That's how quickly I can get sucked back to the dark side of my own head. That's how irrational and powerful these thoughts are. They can momentarily overwrite all of the evidence around me that I am worthwhile, that I am loved, that I have done and continue to do incredible things.

It's estimated that one in every six teens in the U.S. has planned for suicide. In 2017, 10.6 million adults reported having serious thoughts about trying to kill themselves. Even when it feels like it, we're not alone. There are many, many people who struggle with suicidal thoughts every day.

Let me be very clear: **SUICIDE IS NEVER THE ANSWER TO LIFE'S STRUGGLES!** I know how convincing and overpowering these thoughts can sometimes seem. I know that sometimes they can be terrifying, and other times they can seem very reasonable and logical (which is probably even more terrifying).

The majority of people who unsuccessfully attempt suicide do not die from another attempt. Many report being overjoyed that they did not succeed. Life is constantly changing, and whatever situation is overwhelming you right now will change too. This is often hard to keep in mind, especially for people prone to addiction and depression. Our minds can get stuck in the current moment, a distorted reality where the pain we are feeling seems like it will last forever.

I can assure you this is not true. No matter what you are facing or how you are feeling, as long as you are alive, there is a sunny day ahead—a day where the idea of committing suicide seems as impossible as it will ever seem attractive. Even better, you've got a machine that can—well, if not change the weather, at least heavily influence it. You don't have to wait powerlessly for that sunny day.

First off, it's helpful to recognize that suicidal thoughts are closely tied with depression, addiction, and pain—the same elements that we tackle throughout this whole book. The choices that you make to be sober, heal, love, and pursue your passions will help you build a whole arsenal of coping tools. No one has a pain-free life, but one of the many larger benefits of the good choices you're going to make is that you will get stronger and better, but your trauma won't grow. I've had suicidal thoughts in the depths of addiction—living out of my car, so sick, without any sense of love or purpose and a future that no one would have taken bets on—and I have suicidal thoughts now, with an amazing life.

I still have trauma, but I've grown, and it hasn't. It can't push me around the way it used to. Those dark thoughts that tell me I'm worthless have to compete with the many, many parts of myself I've developed, the connections I have formed, and the things in the world I have helped and built that suggest otherwise. When I was surrounded by nothing but my bad choices, I survived my suicidal thoughts with a Hail Mary, last minute pass, a leap of faith that my life could be something more if I just held on. Now, I can train my precision coping skills on those thoughts and prove them wrong pretty quickly. I don't think that side of me will ever go away. But now I have the power to send it away.

Choose to build your physical and emotional strength. Choose to build connections and passions and interests. Understand that

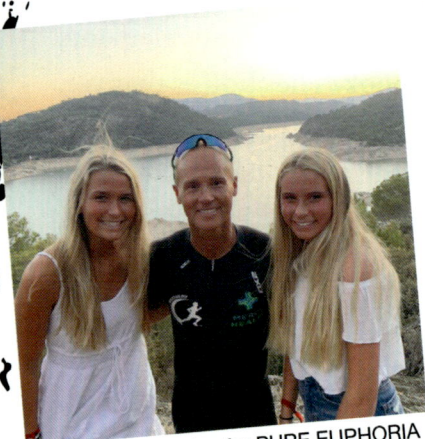
Wrapping up filming for PURE EUPHORIA in Madrid, Spain with my daughters

suicidal thoughts don't mean you want to commit suicide. Consider them alarm bells, like the world's worst smoke detector. Suicidal thoughts are a sign that something is off-balance in your life. Maybe you have something from your past you need to address. (For example, it's probably time to forgive myself for cutting it close to the hospital sixteen years ago; I've learned every lesson that mistake had to teach me long ago.) Maybe it's a signal that you have taken on too much stress, that you're overwhelmed, that you need to make some adjustments. Maybe it's a sign that you need to change something about your nutrition, or sleep schedule, or exercise routine. Choose to use these thoughts to enhance your wellness. You can be an example of how to not only survive suicidal ideation, but how to thrive in life.

There are risk factors for suicidal thoughts that we cannot control—most notably, a genetic predisposition. (On my mom's side of the family, my uncle and aunt also took their own lives.) Find out what your risk factors are, so you can get a head start on treatment.

The most important factors, though, are under your control—even when it doesn't feel like it at all. Having these thoughts does not make you a weak person. Acknowledging them, seeking help, and learning to cope with them will help. Choose healing, choose building, choose understanding yourself better. Suicide is never the right choice.

## SUICIDE STATS

Suicide is the third leading cause of death among adolescents and teenagers. According to the National Institute for Mental Health (NIMH), about 8 out of every 100,000 teenagers committed suicide in 2000. For every teen suicide death, experts estimate there are 10 other teen suicide attempts.

In a survey of high school students, the National Youth Violence

Prevention Resource Center found that almost 1 in 5 teens had thought about suicide, about 1 in 6 teens had made plans for suicide, and more than 1 in 12 teens had attempted suicide in the last year. As many as 8 out of 10 teens who commit suicide try to ask for help in some way before committing suicide, such as by seeing a doctor shortly before the suicide attempt.

Teen girls and boys are both at risk for suicide. Teen girls are more likely to attempt suicide, but teenage boys are four to five times more likely to die by suicide. Over half of teen suicide deaths are inflicted by guns.

**Several factors increase the risk that a teenager will attempt suicide:**

- Depression or feelings of loneliness or helplessness

- Alcohol or drug addiction

- A family history of abuse, suicide, or violence

- Previous suicide attempts; almost half of teens who commit suicide had attempted suicide previously.

- A recent loss such as a death, break-up, or parents' divorce, illness or disability

- Stress over school, relationships, performance expectations, etc.

- Fear of ridicule for getting help for problems

- Being bullied or being a bully

- Exposure to other teens committing suicide, such as at school or in the media

- Access to firearms or other lethal objects

- A belief that suicide is noble

90 percent of people who attempt or commit suicide suffer from a mental illness, such as:

- Depression, which causes a teen to feel sad, lonely, withdrawn, and unable to accomplish simple tasks.

- Bipolar disorder, where a teen alternates between periods of depression and mania, characterized by exuberance, insomnia, irritability, and inability to concentrate.

- Schizophrenia, a complicated condition where a teen has hallucinations or distorted perceptions of reality.

- Alcoholism or drug addiction, especially when combined with another mental health disorder; 20 to 50 percent of suicide attempts are related to drug or alcohol use.

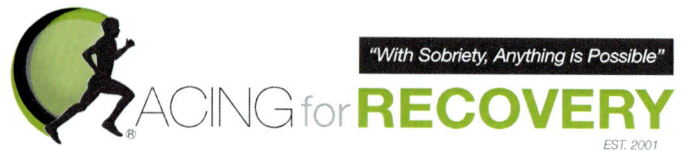

# CHOOSE PASSION

Choosing to heal our bodies and minds prepares us to share our lives with our communities and explore all the gifts we have to offer. When we have reduced the impact of trauma and begin healing, we free ourselves to feel inspired, give back, and help others. You can do incredible things with your life when you're not spending all your time trying to hide from yourself! Once we choose to pursue our passions, our lives become bigger and more meaningful.

## WHAT AM I SUPPOSED TO DO FOR FUN?

I told my parents I was staying at Gary's house. Sometimes that was true, since I knew I could get away with drinking and using drugs there. Other times it wasn't. I'd sleep in the cornfields or in the high school baseball dugout, because I just wanted to drink alone. *Gary is still my best friend.*

I stayed at Bill's one night. His parents were divorced, and his mom let him do whatever he wanted. What I wanted was alcohol and drugs and his Izod alligator shirts, and that's what I got. *Bill died from alcohol and drug issues.*

I also spent many nights at my friend Stacy's, though I don't remember a lot of them. They'd have to carry me into the house and drag me all the way up to his room in the attic. I'd wake up the next morning not remembering a thing. *Stacy died from alcoholism the day I completed IRONMAN Louisville in 2014.*

The party usually started at my place, though. Friends would shimmy up the outside of my house and in my upstairs window. Once we were good and messed up, then we would sneak out. Driving drunk and high to areas where we could continue to party, have sex, and break things.

There was no stopping me during this period in my life. I was determined, and I had no issue with being sneaky or duplicitous. I took advantage of my friends who lacked parental supervision. I took advantage of everyone.

(Madison, my youngest daughter, doesn't get it: "Why would you want to do that? I would rather sleep." Smart kid. She won't end up like me.)

I grew up surrounded by all these good, healthy kids, and I just never felt like I belonged in that group. I started to build walls so that no one else would realize that I was an imposter. Then I found other kids, who were troubled like me.

I had every opportunity, but my pain kept me from being able to see them. I can empathize with people who live in poverty, who come from bad environments, who don't have the access to opportunity that I did, because in my pain, I drove them all away.

Opportunity is only valuable when you're able to use it.

People need two things to succeed: self-esteem and opportunity. If you've got opportunity but no self-esteem, you're not going to be able to use the opportunities. If you've got few opportunities but you have self-esteem, you're going to be able to find opportunities. Even once you've chosen sobriety and healing, it can be hard to know where to turn. When you've built your life around your bad choices, you tend to surround yourself with people and situations that enable or even promote making more bad choices.

I get asked often about how to handle social events and alcohol. One of the first things that I encourage people to ask themselves is why they are going to the event in the first place! Some events offer alcohol, but alcohol isn't the primary purpose for attending, like concerts or sporting events. However, attending a bar, even to see a band, creates an entirely different environment. These are situations that you need to carefully consider putting yourself in. Be realistic about the healing you've done and still have to do in sobriety. If you haven't developed a strong aversion to alcohol, peer pressure, and feeling out of place yet, attending functions with alcohol is a bad idea.

It is unrealistic to live your entire life without being exposed to alcohol. As you become more confident in your sobriety you can expand your exposure. When you can't avoid old environments, you need to pay the closest attention to your actions and think all the way through to their logical conclusions. When you do this, you can recognize behaviors that don't serve your best interests. Attend with a plan. Don't just wing it. If you're at a concert to see the band, or at a birthday to show your friend how much you care, you've got purpose. This goes for attending work parties, weddings, anniversaries, graduations, etc. You'll be better prepared to stay sober after you've thought about the situation and your goals ahead of time.

Develop a network of like-minded friends, and bring along support for social situations where other people may be drinking or using drugs. That way, you can have each other's backs at events. Plan out your escape strategies when you are confronted with situations that will involve drinking.

Choose to avoid alcohol as much as possible. When that isn't an option, make a plan, lean on the support of like-minded people and be honest about your state of mind and potential vulnerability. Don't start looking for signs and excuses to drink. Trust me, when you're the dude that orders water, nine times out of ten, they forget to bring it. (I've noticed the same trend ordering vegan meals—they'll usually remember to leave the chicken off a salad, but there's a 90% chance it'll be covered in cheese.) That's no excuse to abandon your goals. Remember, you are your priority. Applying self-empowering skills and improving your self-esteem is NOT selfish. Taking care of yourself must be your primary goal. Trying to please others, especially at your expense, is a dangerous path to walk. Others will never be as invested in your success as you are. Showing yourself how important you and your health and goals are is great; as a major side benefit, you're also setting an example for the people around you, who might also be struggling.

As you build your new coping skills, it's important to treat yourself right. It is not a good idea to spend time in the same places and with the same people that you used to use around. Everything shouldn't be a test of willpower. Carve out new activities and make new friends who share your goals and lifestyle. Take part in environments and social situations that reflect a sober reality. Many social interactions are based around bars and drinking, so it's easy to feel left out when you're not interested in living like that anymore. It's about looking at the bigger picture and realizing that's not actually connecting you to cooler things in life.

One of the things I've loved most my entire life is music. My dad said that by the time I was two and a half, I could work his record player. When he took me to nursery school for the first time, there was this nursery rhyme stuff playing.

I looked at the teacher. "Um, you guys got any Beatles?"

The teacher looked surprised. "No."

"You got any Creedence Clearwater Revival?"

"No."

"You got any Zeppelin?"

"No."

I looked at my dad. "I'm out of here, I don't want to do it."

I can't tell you how many concerts I was so excited about seeing when I was struggling that I can't remember at all. I used enough drugs and alcohol to completely blackout my experience.

I still listen to music throughout every day. It's just a natural part of what I do. It helps me get through difficult times, and it helps me celebrate good times. I wake up at 4:30 to some meditation music, but it gets louder as time goes on. I run to it, I do yoga to it, it motivates me to do IRONMAN, to deal with emotions effectively. Listening to music sober is a completely different mindset. Songs that I used to listen to when I was drunk that would make me more depressed are a relief now, cathartic, and stir up memories of overcoming and triumphing. It's just this total cognitive shift.

Now, when I attend concerts, I can fully enjoy the shows and remember them. By choosing to pursue my passion, I've also been able to connect my love of music with helping people and reaching out for support.

I love taking people from Racing for Recovery to see bands. One week this spring, I took three guys to Metallica on Monday in Indianapolis, then two girls and one guy to KISS Wednesday in Detroit. We did Metallica in Cleveland and Pittsburgh, Tesla in Chicago and Detroit, and a few Motley Crue shows sprinkled in. I don't try to label it as art or music therapy (although we often find it is). I just want to chill with them and show them how

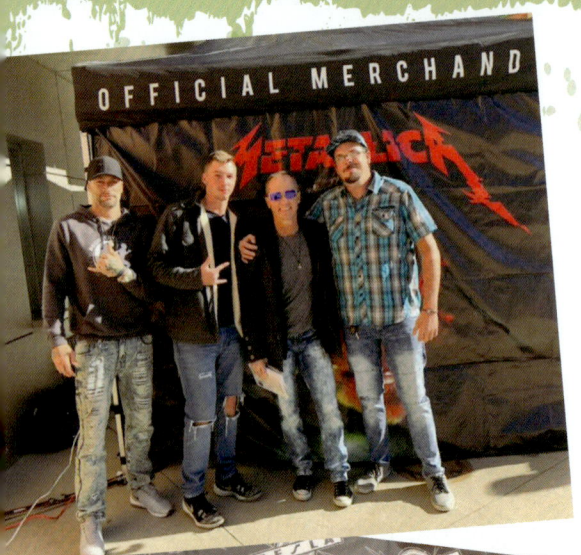

awesome life in recovery can be. When I take new people to do these types of things, they start to experience the extreme upsides to choosing the right things, and it motivates them to keep improving their lives. It's great just to watch people understand themselves better and get to experience some of these cool things.

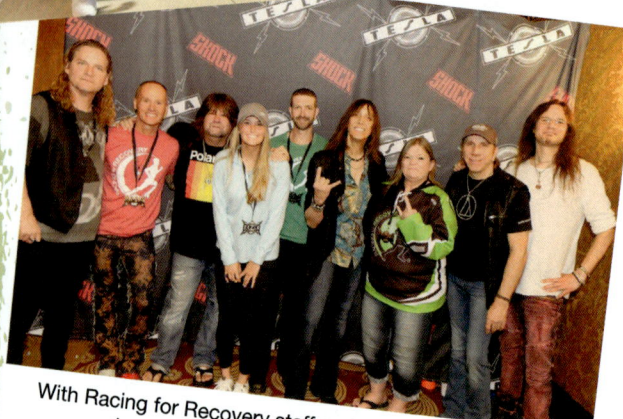

With Racing for Recovery staff and peers along with my daughter Skylar at Metallica and TESLA

One guy I've recently connected with in recovery had been in prison for sixteen of his fifty-two years. He's battled drugs for forty years. He doesn't trust anybody.

"Hey man, do you want to go to Metallica?"

"I don't have any money."

"That's not what I asked."

People aren't used to being treated well, so it's my job to help build the trust. When we were walking into the arena, he told me, "I started to realize you brought me here because you like me as a person. That touched me so much."

I was looking for a cool way to celebrate the twenty-sixth anniversary of when I chose sobriety, and I realized that Aerosmith was doing a residency out in Vegas. I marched right into group therapy.

"Hey, write down your top three bands."

I found two people who love their music, who'd been utilizing what Racing for Recovery offers and doing the work. I wanted them to be blown away, to have a lifetime memory, so that when it gets hard, they can look back on it and use some of the strength they felt that night to carry on in their sobriety and achieve their goals. So we went and saw Aerosmith together in Las Vegas—we even got to sit on stage with them and meet them!

I just took three guys to Chicago to meet and see Tesla in this old theater. We had our own private booth overlooking the stage, and we were probably the only ones in the crowd not drinking. While the band was playing, we watched a girl puke on the bar across the way.

After the show, I texted my friend in the band, and he came up to our booth. My three guys were a little starstruck at first, but very quickly realized he's just a regular guy.

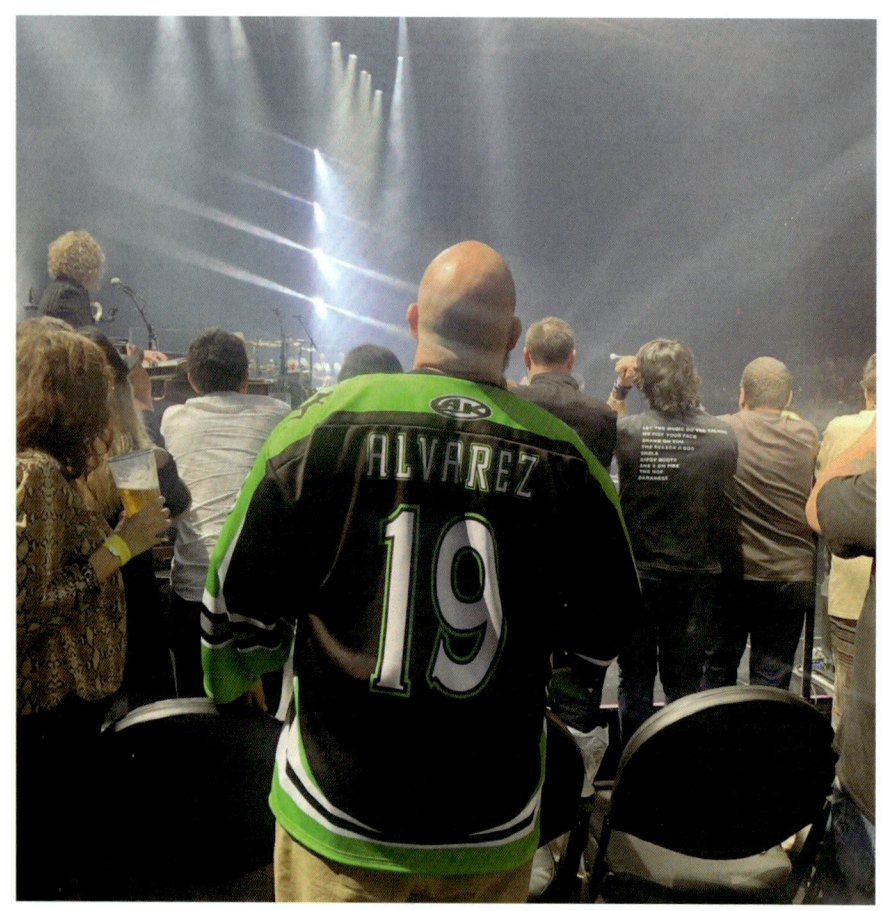

Racing for Recovery success story Bobby Alzarez in his jersey on stage with Aerosmith in Las Vegas 2019

"Dave, did you see the chick puking on the bar during your set?"

He started to laugh. "No, I missed that. I find it really strange that someone would pay all this money to come and get that drunk and not remember us playing."

We didn't feel out of place; we felt bad for everyone else there, who was diluting this awesome experience with drinking. We were just four guys who liked each other, liked this band, who were thinking in a positive manner and wanted to enjoy the music. It's a pretty big bonus, that, because of who we are and what we're committed to, we get to meet up with the band and hang out. Everyone else in the crowd could only wish they were having the same type of night.

**CHOOSING PASSION MEANS MORE THAN JUST MANAGING YOUR ENVIRONMENT. YOU'RE NOT DOOMED TO A LIFE OF LESS THAN—DOING EVERYTHING YOU WERE DOING BEFORE, JUST MINUS DRUGS AND ALCOHOL. YOU ARE CAPABLE OF DOING, BEING, AND SEEING SO MUCH MORE IN SOBRIETY THAN YOU EVER COULD HAVE WHEN YOU WERE STRUGGLING WITH ADDICTION.**

Get out there and start doing the things you're passionate about, and recognize all the opportunities to make them bigger and better and cooler now that you're sober. Drugs and alcohol limited you from experiencing things you loved—there are no limits anymore. Choose passion and make things happen.

It's an incredible experience, meeting and getting to know people who are sober, who value sobriety around them, and who are also some of the biggest rock stars the world has ever seen. When I realized how many of the musicians I grew up idolizing struggled with alcohol and drugs too, I felt a true bond to them. I was shocked to find out the feelings were mutual.

So many of my musical heroes have gone out of their way to get the Racing for Recovery message out into the world. The first time I heard Tesla, I was drinking at our local swimming quarry. Now I know them, we're friends, and their music is featured in our second and third documentaries. Bret Michaels' first solo record runs through our whole first documentary; he charged me ten cents a song. Blas Elias, drummer for Burning Rain, who was not only the lead drummer for the band Slaughter and part of the famous Blue Man

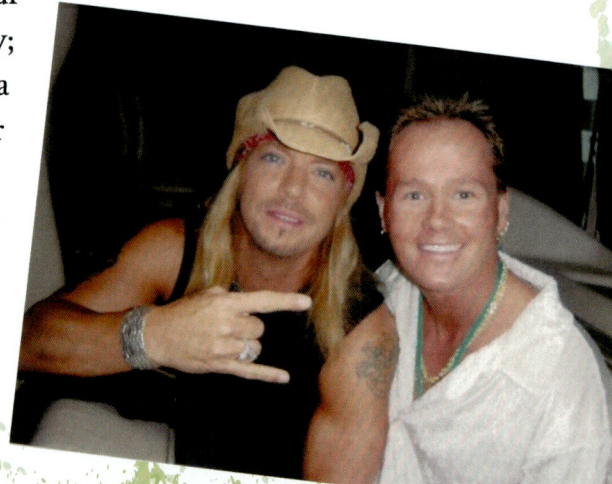

Group, but also tours with the Trans-Siberian Orchestra, has supported Racing for Recovery for years.

I give out Racing for Recovery hockey jerseys whenever I meet a musician who has struggled with drugs and alcohol and inspires others to find sobriety. Stephen Tyler and Joe Perry from Aerosmith thought they were awesome; I'm looking forward to seeing them again in November and handing them copies of this book and our newest documentary. Poison got their jerseys in Toronto. I've hung out with them backstage a bunch of times, so I felt pretty bold.

"Bret, can you wear this tonight?"

Bret Michaels shook his head and said kindly, "Nah, man, I really can't, I'm used to wearing this. I've got to be comfortable to perform right."

I didn't even have time to be a little disappointed before Rikki Rockett piped up, "I'll wear it."

So,

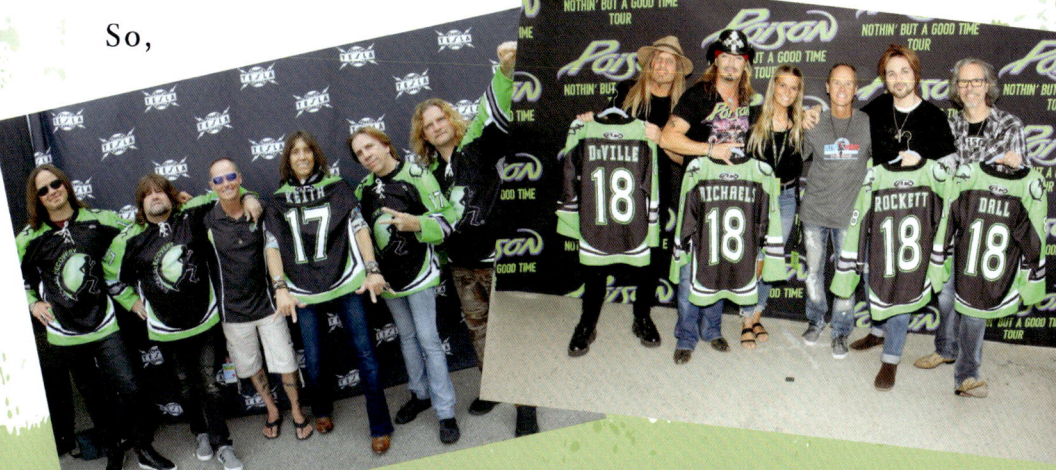

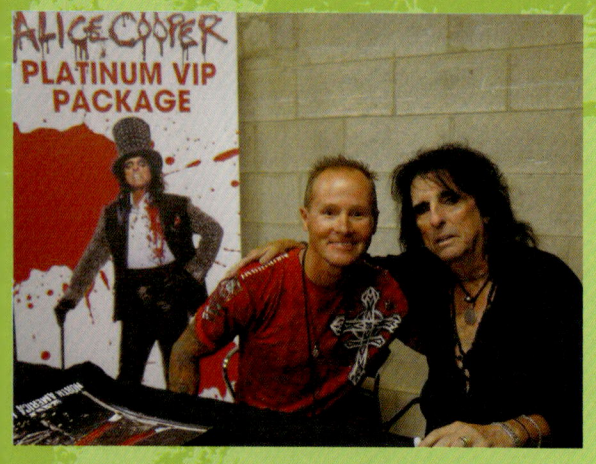

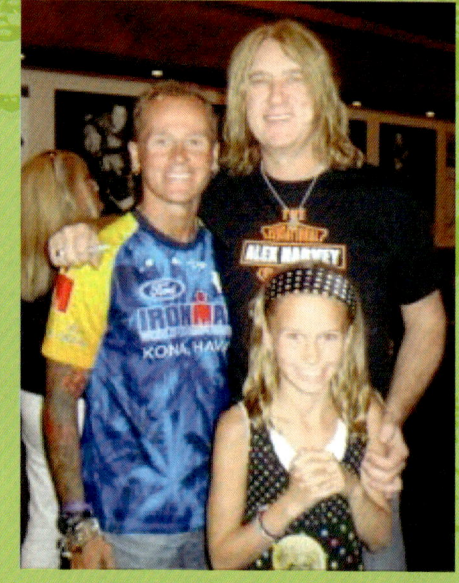

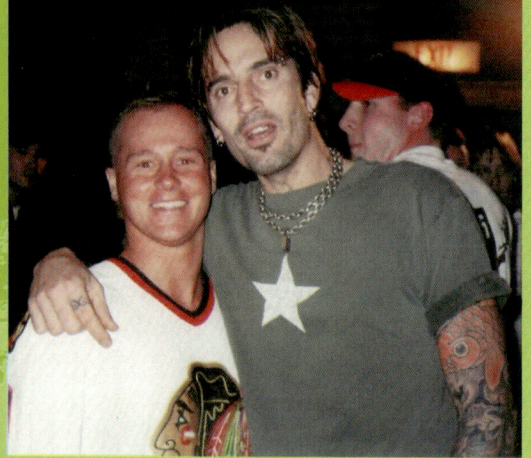

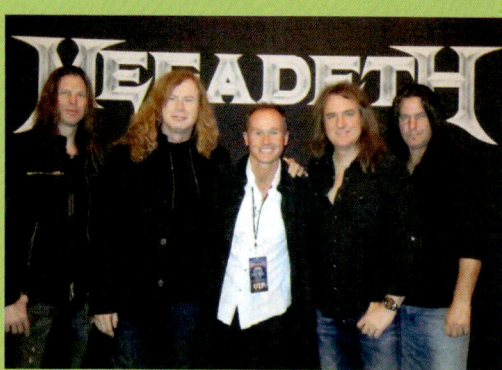

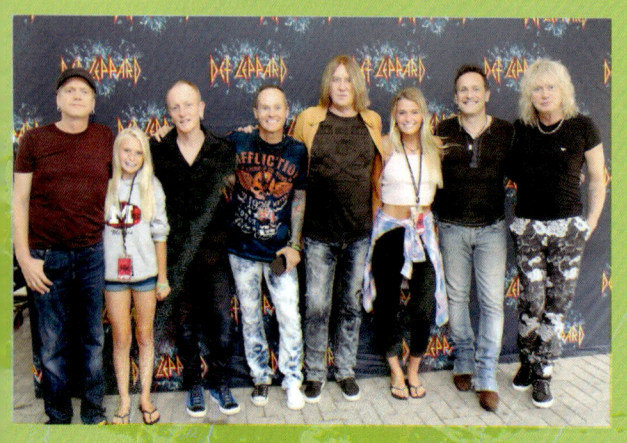

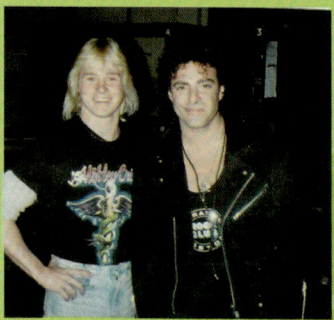

This page clockwise from top left: with Alice Cooper; with my daughter Skylar and Joe Elliot from Def Leppard; with Megadeath; with Neal Schon from Journey; with my daughters Skylar and Madison and Def Leppard; with Tommy Lee from Motley Crue

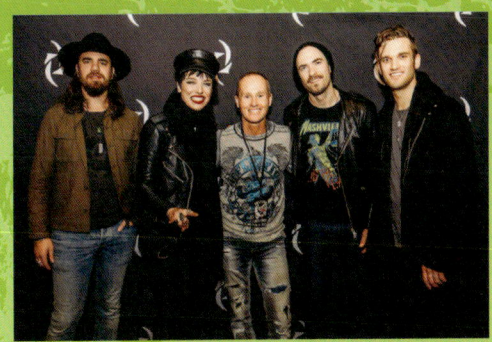

Halestorm

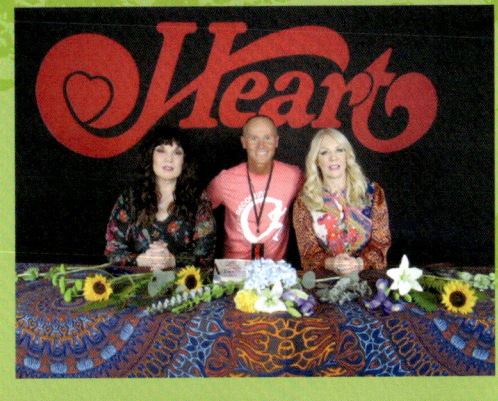

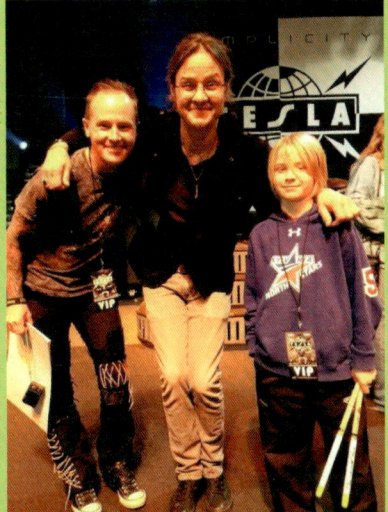

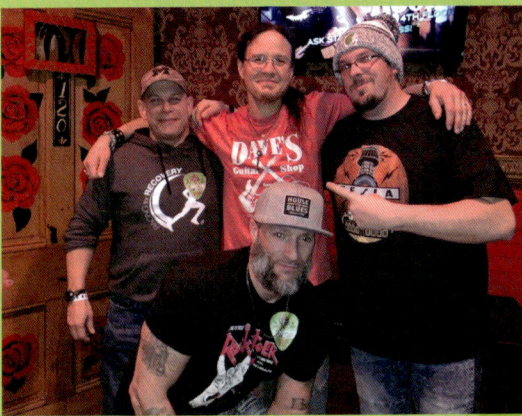

Peers and myself with Dave Rude from TESLA

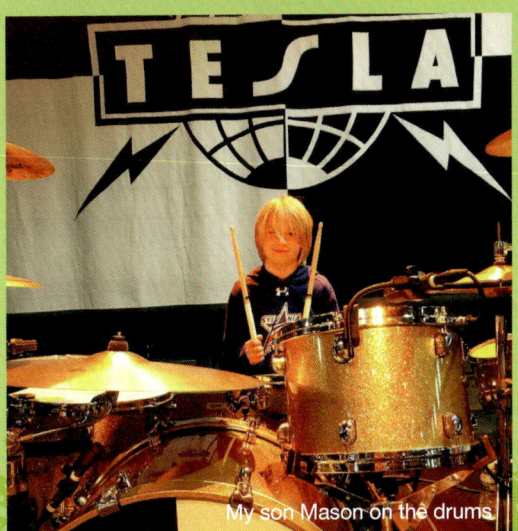

My son Mason on the drums

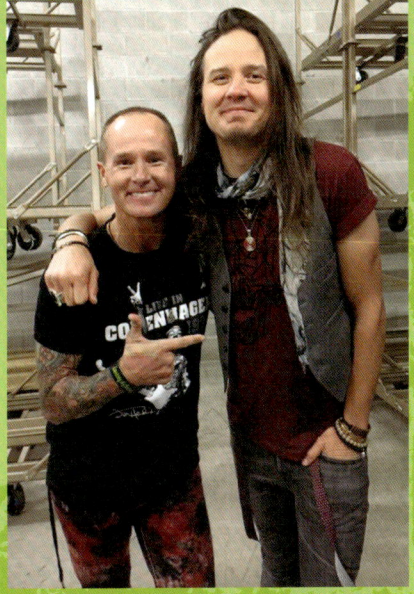

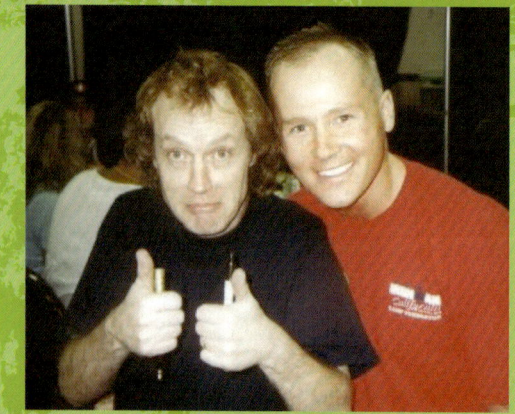

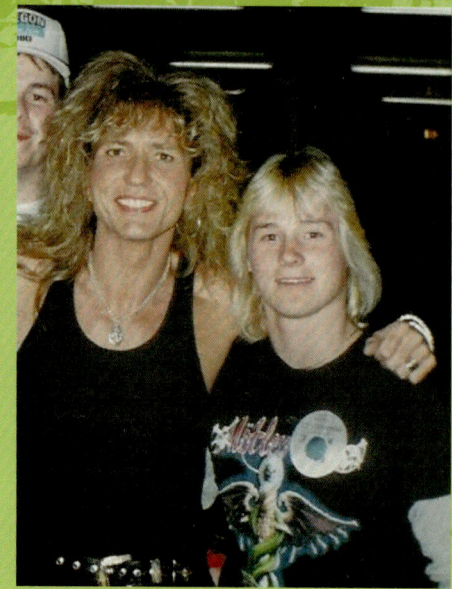

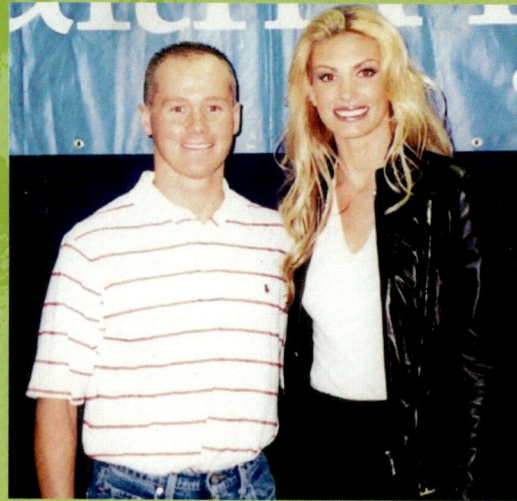

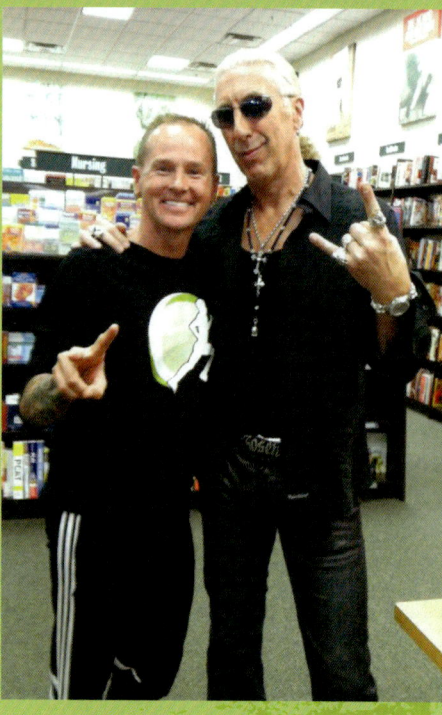

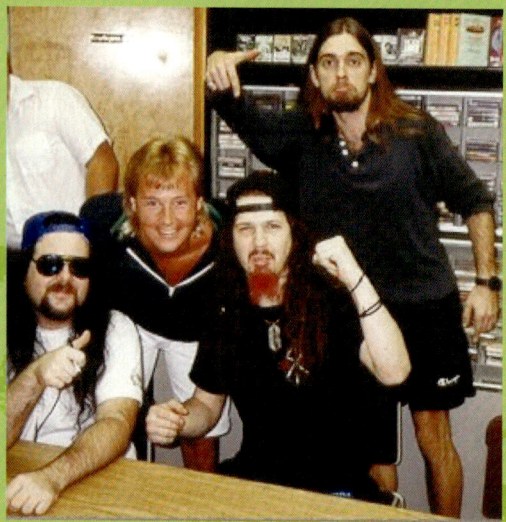

This page clockwise from top left: with Angus Young of AC/DC; with David Coverdale of Whitesnake (back in the hair days); with Dee Snider of Twisted Sister; with Pantera; and with Faith Hill

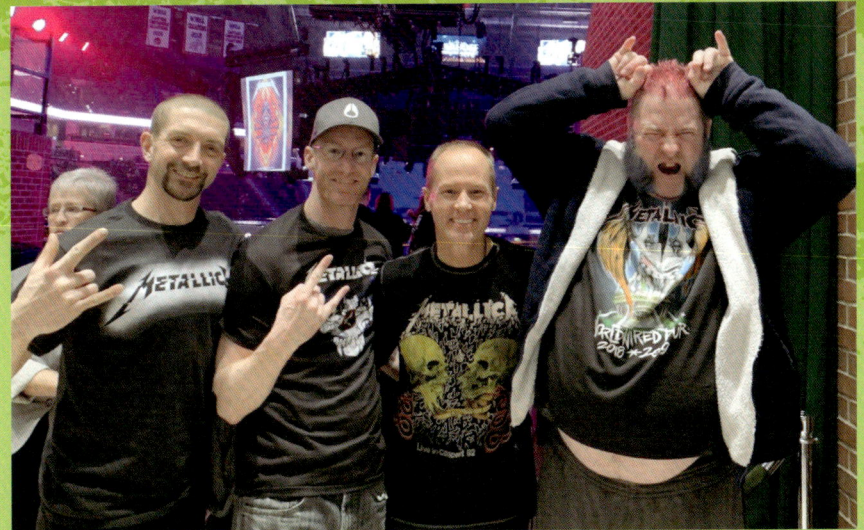

This page: at Metallica concert with Racing for Recovery friends; with Metallica band members; and Metallica receiving their Racing for Recovery jerseys

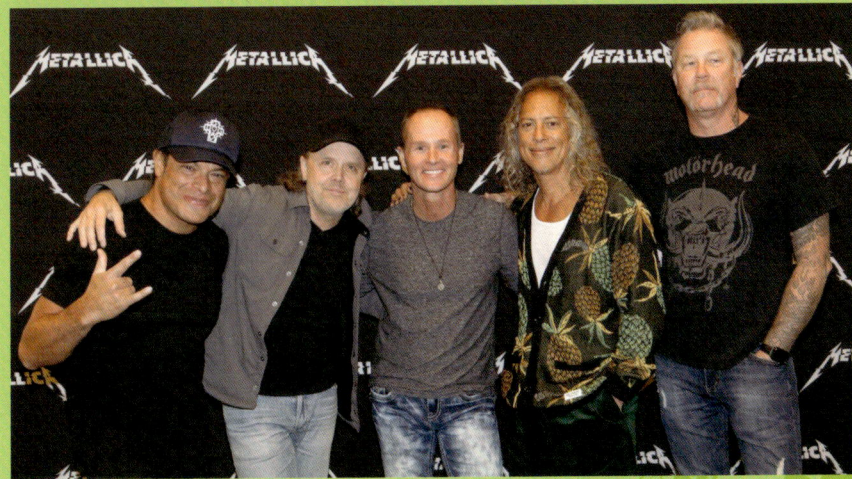

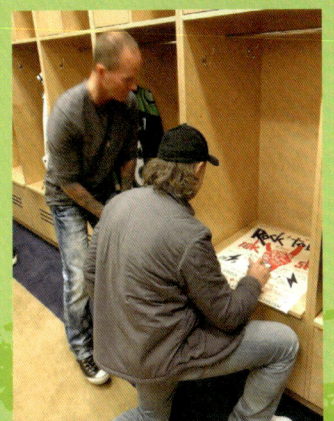

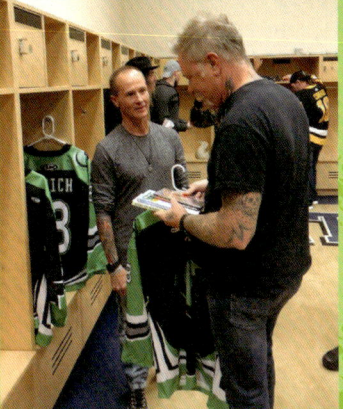

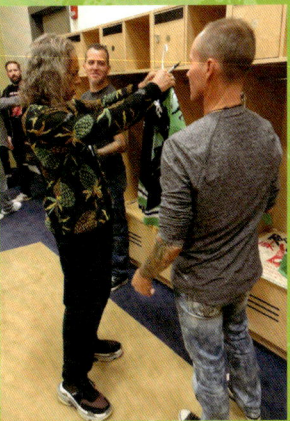

there's a YouTube video of one of the best rock drummers in the world wearing a Racing for Recovery jersey on stage.

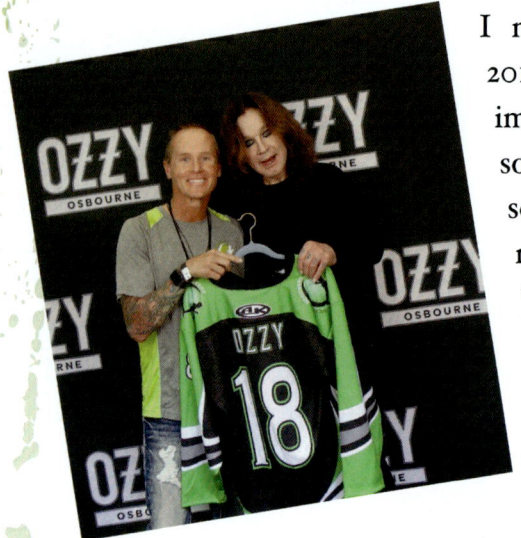

I met Ozzy in the summer of 2018, and we talked about how important exercise is for our sobriety (as I recall, it went something like, "Todd, if I don't ride my bike every day, I go *#%! CRAZY!"). I took my son Mason backstage to meet Motley Crue, and I told Nikki Sixx what I was up to with Racing for Recovery. He was shocked.

I could go on for pages and pages about all of the powerful, inspiring interactions I've had with rock stars since I chose sobriety, but I think I've got enough to illustrate the point: Cool people who do cool things encourage and support other cool people who are doing cool things.

It's not selfish to choose to pursue your passions—not even a little bit! When you're pursuing things you're passionate about, you encourage the people around you to pursue their favorite activities. This strengthens them emotionally and instills them with self-worth, and teaches you a lot about yourself. Who do you care enough about to step away from your own pain to help them find happiness? What gives you energy? What do you enjoy showing people and teaching them? What type of help can you offer that fills you up, rather than depleting your strength?

Because of who I am and what I do, I hear a lot of dreams that people assume they've lost forever: "God, I really wanted to be a chef one day," "I always thought I would be a personal trainer," "I wanted to use my art to help people." I can look each of these people in the eye and tell them to get their acts together and use the resources all around us. Racing for Recovery has a kitchen, a gym, classrooms and presentation spaces, and we will do anything to encourage dreams.

Learning the difference between your needs when you're making the wrong decisions and your needs when you're making good choices can take time. People who've struggled with addiction can feel guilty, like we've already used our quotas of time and resources. Doing things for yourself can feel selfish; it can seem unfair to invest in yourself until you've given back to the people and the world that you hurt with your choices in addiction. I'm not immune to that type of thinking, even in sobriety. I'll never forget when I was at IRONMAN Quebec and got the phone call that my son Konor had broken both his wrists. Melissa had been at work, and I was in Canada, and Konor had constructed a zipline. His brothers had both zipped down, but when Konor got on, it snapped, and he plummeted about twenty feet. I felt so guilty that I hadn't been there. I was ready to hop on the first plane back, but Melissa stopped me and pointed out that I wouldn't be able to help. Not doing the race, the thing that was bringing attention to my life's purpose and helping people attain sobriety, wasn't going to heal Konor's wrists. Choosing not to do something you're passionate about out of solidarity for someone else in a bad spot isn't a good choice.

I've never met a more caring, loving, intelligent, artistic, and kind group of people than those who have suffered from addiction. It never ceases to amaze me how willing hurting people are to do anything for anyone. The problem is that they don't give themselves the same love, care, and generosity. They freely give to others, but they have trouble believing they deserve to give themselves anything.

**YOU CANNOT BELIEVE THAT. POINT BLANK. THERE IS NOTHING SELFISH ABOUT HEALING. THERE IS NOTHING SELFISH ABOUT PURSUING YOUR PASSIONS. THERE IS NOTHING SELFISH ABOUT MAKING YOURSELF A BETTER PERSON.**

I struggled a lot with this (which we will discuss more in when we're looking at choosing love). I knew, from the very bottom of my soul, that Racing for Recovery was my life's purpose. I knew that the races I ran were helping people in pain find help. I knew I deserved to be happy. I knew I had to keep doing it, even when it was costing me everything.

Once I let go of the idea that choosing my passion made me selfish, I was able to use the gifts I was building in all areas of my life. It wasn't compartmentalized to my dream. My dreams made me a better father, husband, son, friend—my dreams made me a bigger and better person.

Do you know what I've noticed about dreams? They're only selfish if you don't do them. Here, try to think of a single dream that's selfish if you're really working to make it happen. A chef creates amazing meals for other people. A trainer makes other people stronger and healthier. An artist helps people understand things they haven't been able to express. Running an IRONMAN is incredible, but the best part about it is watching how it affects the people around you, seeing the glimmer in their eyes when they realize that anything is possible—that they can do the impossible too.

I work with a very intelligent, kind, and compassionate young man who also happens to be one heck of a swimmer. He has struggled over the years with substance abuse and self-value. In one of our recent individual counseling sessions, he said, "Things are not happening in sobriety as quickly or how I thought they would be. I need to find value in myself."

That hit my heart. I wished I could show him how incredible

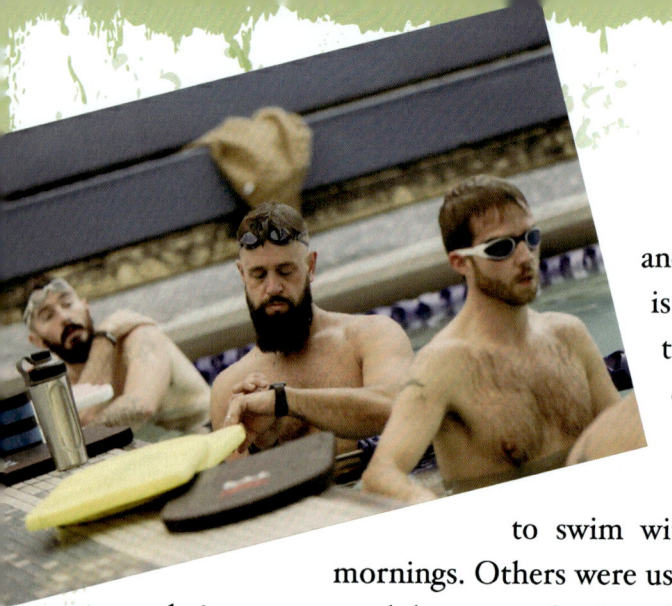

and valuable I think he is, but it doesn't work that way. Instead, I encouraged him to start swimming again and invited him to swim with us on Wednesday mornings. Others were using exercise as part of their recovery, and they wanted to learn how to swim. I learned how to swim to compete in IRONMAN—teaching others is above my skill level!

The very first morning, he showed up at 5:30 AM and made a huge difference in the lives of the five people who wanted to swim. He used his gifts and talents and passions and helped other people overcome obstacles. He even gave me some pointers that have helped me in several IRONMAN races since. We were all grateful for the ways he shared and helped and made us stronger, and he could see those results. He was building self-worth, one step at a time, learning to value the incredible things he was capable of, by creating change in the world around him.

In therapy, we focus on telling your story. It's important to craft your story and become the hero. No one else is going to save you; we just can't. You become the hero by making the right choices, by pursuing the right paths. When you become the hero, you realize you have an unending supply of inspiration and greatness inside of you, and you're eager to make it matter. I still have trouble accepting that I'm the hero of my story sometimes, which is why I work on projects like this book. Sometimes, I would love to hide out (it's the darker side of insisting I'm the janitor around here). I know that I'm prone to feeling useless and worthless, and I know those feelings don't help me or anyone else in my life. I do whatever I can to make sure I'm doing great things, so I see the greatness inside of me reflected in what I build and do and who I help.

If you're looking for a passion that's all about you, you're never going to find it. Surrounding yourself with stuff doesn't work—it's not your life's purpose. When you find your life's passion, I guarantee you that it's going to involve helping other people. If you're not quite sure yet what yours is, get a head start by helping others and encouraging them. The self-worth that you build and the inspiration you get will guide you towards the path you're supposed to pursue.

## WHY ISN'T THIS STUFF MAKING ME HAPPY?

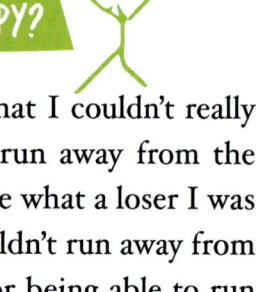

I sat in my apartment, so high and drunk that I couldn't really get up. That sucked, because I wanted to run away from the voice inside my head that just kept telling me what a loser I was and how I didn't deserve to be alive. If I couldn't run away from that voice, I probably would have settled for being able to run away from the guy on the other side of the room looking through my CD collection. He wouldn't stop telling me how awesome I was...because I had a nice stereo. Because I had a lot of CDs. I hated him for falling for it. I hated myself for not being able to.

Totally unfair, because I'd set the trap. I'd bought that stereo, and all those CDs, so that people would think I was awesome, even after I'd realized that it wouldn't make me feel awesome. I wanted the best of everything. I wanted to look good. I wanted to be somebody.

When I was a kid, I went to good schools. I lived in a nice new housing development. I had many friends. I had God-given athletic ability. I wore nice clothes. I had all the bikes, skateboards, and sports equipment that any kid could ever ask for. It was a nice little package on the outside, but I went home every night thinking about killing myself. You can wrap a box up like the most beautiful gift in the world, but it doesn't change what's inside. I just kept putting more bows on a box full of turds.

I felt like a turd inside, all the time. I hated feeling that way, but I didn't think I had any other choice—how could you not feel like a turd if you are a turd? It scared me a lot to think that other people would see how awful I was. Before I ever picked up my first drink, I started trying to hide who I thought I was, so no one else would notice. Even though my stuff was valuable (or at least expensive), it didn't increase my value. Some people were impressed sometimes, but most people weren't. I wasn't. I was still lost, hopeless, lonely, isolated, suicidal, and sad.

It was mind-blowing to be around people who had self-esteem and used their money and things the way they were meant to be used. They wore the clothes that made them feel comfortable and that they could do the things they loved to do in. They had the CDs of music that they just enjoyed listening to, because it made their already full lives even richer. It was even weirder when someone had little, but somehow seemed to be happy. I just couldn't ever feel that way.

There was nothing wrong with the toys, bikes, clothes and equipment my loving parents and grandparents gave me. The problem was internal, and no amount of "stuff" could solve my emotional problems. The stuff I had just highlighted my depression and my sense of worthlessness. The worse I felt, the more I wanted to medicate. The more I medicated, the worse I felt. All the stuff I had became symbols of what I didn't deserve and amplified my negative emotions.

Very few people who struggle with the type of pain that leads to choosing drugs and alcohol only choose drugs and alcohol. We usually have many things that we try to fill the holes in ourselves with—excessive spending, gambling, sex, food, stuff. Even people who never turn to drugs and alcohol can fall into the trap of thinking they can use outside things to heal inside. The things they choose often fly under the radar, and they might even get a lot of praise for how much effort they put into their external coping mechanisms—dressing nicely, getting good grades, overachieving in their lives. If they don't learn to love themselves and pursue their passions, however pretty their lives might look from the outside, they'll still feel like a box of turds on the inside.

It's important to understand where happiness comes from. It's a hard lesson to learn! We live in a world driven by materialism. When we're little kids, we're taught to value our "stuff" before we learn to value ourselves. When we get good grades, we get rewarded. When we behave ourselves, we get rewarded. It's hard to teach us the "whys" of our choices before we start stacking up the consequences, which means we get weird messages. Our brains make the connection that when we get a good grade, people around us are proud and love us. We don't understand that the reason they are proud and love us is because of who we are, and that their happiness over our grades runs deeper than that "A." They don't explain to us that the reason that "A" makes them happy is because they want us to have full, rich lives, and that taking advantage of the opportunities around us can set us up for more success.

Actually, they might not even know it themselves! It's easy to get bogged down in the details and lose sight of the bigger picture: Nothing you can choose to collect, from good grades to nice shirts to big houses, is going to make or break you. "Stuff" will come and go in your life, even when you make all the right choices. The work that you do to build self-value helps you choose the right thing so that you're always building and growing, even when your collection of "stuff" looks bleak. People equate "stuff" and money with happiness. People who don't have these things feel like they are missing out, but people who acquire these things realize this wasn't the answer.

It can be even harder for people working on rebuilding their lives in sobriety to understand this. We've spent so much time in image-management mode that we don't even realize we need to break the habit. We start feeling good about ourselves because we start making the right choices, and we want our outsides to reflect that, STAT. We're concerned with showing everyone else that we're better.

Know the game whack-a-mole, where you have to keep smashing

the head of the mole, no matter which hole he comes out of? In early recovery, if you're not addressing your underlying emotional issues, all the energy that you put towards your addiction might come out in a new outlet. This can be particularly hard to see as a problem when drugs or alcohol abuse are replaced with socially acceptable behaviors, like working obsessively or building up the material stuff that we think successful people have. There really isn't a substitute to looking inward and dealing with the wounds which trigger compulsive behaviors.

I have some version of this conversation every day:

"Hey Todd, I'm thinking about going back to work."

"Why?"

"I need the money."

"Did you make some money while you were struggling with alcohol and drugs?"

"Well, yeah..."

"Were you working before you came into Racing for Recovery?"

"Yes."

"Did drugs and alcohol play a role in you losing your job and your money?"

"Yes."

"Did money and work keep you from using drugs and alcohol?"

"No."

"Have you learned everything you need to know about never using drugs and alcohol again?"

"Not even close."

"There's your answer. If you haven't healed from some of the crap that brought you in here, a freaking job's not gonna fix that."

I get it. I failed at that too. I was sober and I had a beautiful family and a great job, but I didn't like my life or myself. Until I chose to pursue my passions, until I chose to believe in my own intrinsic value, until I decided I deserved to be happy and I was good enough to make the world a better place, those holes inside of me couldn't heal.

Choosing passion is about realizing that all those outside things aren't significant, and you're not going to feel significant just for stacking them up.

I'll never forget pulling into the parking lot of my old office at the same time as my client. We parked next to each other, and he hopped out of a gleaming work truck, probably worth sixty or eighty thousand dollars. He pointed towards my twelve-year-old

Subaru and kind of smirked.

"Dude, you drive that?"

That would have crushed me when I was younger. I would have come up with any excuse in the book to explain it away. Instead, I felt a flood of relief when I said, "Yeah, man—no car payment!"

That's the truth. At the time, I couldn't afford to drive a great car and choose my passion. That wasn't anything to be ashamed of—in fact, it made me proud. There never has been and never will be a car worth more than waking up every day to heal myself and help other people.

## WHAT IF I LOSE EVERYTHING?

Starting Racing for Recovery was a huge turning point in my life. I'd found my purpose, my passion. I wasn't embarrassed anymore by the choices I'd made and the things I'd done—I wasn't proud of all of them, but I was moving forward. I was engaging with the world around me as myself, flaws and all. It was scary, but it was awesome. I felt better than I had in my entire life.

I was playing in the hockey arena with my buddies and my three-year-old son when my best friend rushed over to me.

"Todd, they're taking your car."

I scooped up my son and ran outside. He was right. They were repossessing my car. I couldn't pay for it, and they were taking it back.

My buddy and I ran around, getting the stuff out of the car, getting the car seat out. I tallied this loss up with the foreclosure notices on the house. I'd gone to putt at the Racing for Recovery golf benefit on the phone with the electric company, literally begging them not to turn our lights off. I don't care who you are or how much self-worth you've got—that doesn't feel great.

"Daddy, why are they taking our car?"

I looked at my son and answered: "Because I don't want it anymore."

As soon as the words were out of my mouth, I realized they were true.

The car, the house—even the electric—that was stuff. It was nice stuff to have, but I wanted more. I wanted passion. I wanted to pursue my life's purpose. If it was a choice between that stuff and making the difference I knew I'd been set on this earth to make—well, then I didn't want that stuff anymore.

**OF COURSE, IT WAS HARD! OF COURSE, IT WAS STRESSFUL!** I had four kids! I live in Ohio—it's not like we could have stuck it out camping in the woods for a year or two! But I knew I wanted a different type of life; I knew I deserved it. I knew my kids deserved to grow up seeing and knowing that it was possible, because a lot of things in life would tell them it wasn't. I'd chosen to pursue my passion. If it was easy and safe, it wouldn't be a hard choice to make.

**WHEN YOU CHOOSE TO PURSUE YOUR LIFE'S PASSION, YOUR SOBRIETY, YOUR HEALING, AND YOUR LIFE TAKE TOP PRIORITY. LOSING "STUFF" JUST DOESN'T MATTER AS MUCH TO YOU; IT CERTAINLY DOESN'T THREATEN THE CHOICES YOU MAKE OR THE PERSON YOU'RE COMMITTED TO BECOMING. IT CAN BE STRESSFUL, BUT IT DOESN'T THREATEN YOUR SOBRIETY OR YOUR COMMITMENT TO YOUR GOALS. YOU SEE OPPORTUNITY EVERYWHERE, EVEN IN LOSS. YOU'RE NEVER A VICTIM.**

New Year's Eve, 2017, somebody stole the Racing for Recovery van. If I didn't understand where that ranked in my life's purpose, I probably would have been really discouraged: we need that van, why do bad things happen to nice organizations, I'm just trying to help, blah blah whatever.

Instead, I got on the news and offered free treatment to the person who made the bad decision to take the van.

He hadn't taken away a valuable resource—he'd given us an opportunity to reach out and help more people. He gave us a news story that got traction and got our name out there during

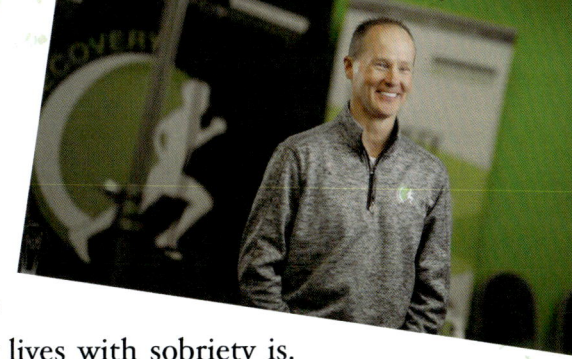

one of the hardest times of the year for a lot of people. That van wasn't my life's purpose; helping people build new, balanced, healthy lives with sobriety is. There isn't any "stuff" I can lose that impacts that passion.

Choosing passion is about realizing what you're willing to do when you believe in your purpose and your future. I lost everything to keep this going, and now I have everything I've ever dreamed of. I'm not talking materialistic stuff. Yes, I have some nice things, but I have fulfilled my life's purpose. You can't put a price tag on that.

## SO, WHAT'S THE DIFFERENCE BETWEEN PASSION AND "POSITIVE" ADDICTION?

Years before I took my first drink, I felt abandoned, hopeless, confused, worthless, hurt, angry, and lost. Athletics, particularly hockey, were my saving grace. On the ice or on the field, I felt secure, content, confident, at peace, and valuable.

By the time I was in sixth grade, I was playing on two different hockey teams, a baseball team, and a soccer team, all at the same time. I played every moment that I wasn't in school or in bed. My dad thought it was a little too much, but I thought it was just enough to keep me focused and entertained. I didn't give myself space to feel bad.

Unfortunately, the Band-Aid wasn't sufficient for a wound that needed open heart surgery. When I wasn't playing sports, I was still overwhelmed by the despair I felt inside. Sports helped distract me, but I wasn't fixing the emotional trauma or healing my pain—I was merely covering it up. When I found drugs and alcohol, I found another way to numb the pain. Athletics or alcohol, I wasn't going to discriminate—whatever I had to do to not feel this way, I was going to do.

I can't tell you the number of times I heard that I'd traded one addiction for another when I started competing in IRONMAN. Seemed believable to me! After all, athletics had been my first coping mechanism. And if I could use my "positive addiction" to stay sober and inspire others, well, that was pretty cool, right?

But something about it just never sat right. For one, there was a six-year lag between choosing sobriety and when I started racing, so calling it a trade seemed weird. There was also something very different about how athletics had functioned in my life as a kid and what role they filled now.

In 2006, I ran the Boston Marathon, and my publicist tagged

along for my tv and radio interviews. For one of the first times, I really opened up about some of my troubles with the story that I'd traded drugs for running. The conversations we had reshaped my understanding.

Addiction controls your life. There's no such thing as a "positive addiction," and thinking about my running in those terms wasn't helping me, because it didn't encourage me to consider how my exercise needed to be in balance in my life. Addictions are out-of-balance; they take over other parts of your life and set your schedule and determine your needs. They compel your behavior. I wasn't pursuing a healthy and productive lifestyle compulsively; I was working to balance different aspects of my life with my new focus. Being athletic and fit is a gift, and with that gift, I have been able to give back through my organization and inspiration. I know that when someone I work with completes a triathlon or marathon or any major goal, I don't dismiss or belittle it as a transference of their addiction. It is an accomplishment, and it helps with all of the aspects of recovery.

I chose drugs and alcohol because I had little self-worth. Accomplishing things like triathlons helped me build self-worth and pursue my passions. I was racing for recovery, not merely in recovery and doing some things like races.

Running is the best mental, emotional, and physical release and overall enhancement I've incorporated into my life in sobriety.

There is nothing wrong with that. Anything that helps someone stay focused and healthy is a good thing. For a person who had no self-worth and had yet to find life's purpose, finding IRONMAN and forming Racing for Recovery started to help me heal and build the skills to fill that emotional void. I wasn't using it to cover over that hole—I was using it to make myself stronger and better, so that I could create a balanced, healthy, sober life.

When someone in a group once asked for the distinction between my addictive behavior with drugs and alcohol and my behavior with endurance racing, I think my buddy Dan may have said it best: "I did a lot of drugs with Todd; the difference was that dude didn't want to live." That's just it. When I was struggling with addiction, I wasn't partying. I was pouring it in like I didn't want to wake up the next morning—because I didn't.

Honestly, there was a period between 2006 and 2009 where I went over the top with triathlons. I knew that my message was hitting home with people, and races helped bring attention to my method of treating addiction, so I was bound and determined to do as many races as I could. All of those races took a toll on my body and my mind, and by 2009, I was toast. I was torturing myself with physical exercise, when I didn't care whether I had a heart attack. I wasn't healed. I wasn't in balance. I wasn't using a "positive addiction." I was hurting myself, and I chose whether I was going to heal and pursue my passions, or whether I was going to pursue addiction. I couldn't have both.

I had to take a good look at why I'd started doing triathlons in the first place and start living more in balance. Finding balance has been an interesting, educational, and life-changing experience. Now, I can tell people confidently that exercise isn't a "positive addiction." It is part of a balanced life. When we're working towards keeping our lives in balance—choosing sobriety, healing, and passion through our academics, work, faith, community, and other activities—then we're happy, confident, and well-rounded. We're experiencing everything life has to offer. **CHOOSING PASSION IS ABOUT BEING IN BALANCE AND UNDERSTANDING THAT NO ONE ELEMENT CAN TAKE OVER YOUR LIFE. WHEN ANYTHING (NO MATTER HOW "GOOD" THAT THING IS, STARTS DISTURBING YOUR BALANCE, IT'S NO LONGER A PASSION— IT'S A PROBLEM.**

Often, people will say, I have an addictive personality. Choosing passion means recognizing that this type of thinking dismisses the amazing things you can do! As we heal, we learn things that add to our health, fitness, nutrition, academics, joy, success, and relationships—things that are great, that make our lives incredible. So...why wouldn't we dive into them? I do things with 100 percent commitment and effort. I value hard work, tenacity, and dedication. I was just as committed to my addiction as I now am to my sobriety, but that is not a character flaw or an expression of my addiction. That's part of what makes me great.

In 1993, I decided I was going to kill myself. I spent three days running around, trying to work up the courage to just do it. In the end, I just couldn't. There was some passion inside of me that was pulling me in another direction. I had no clue what it was, but I spontaneously chose sobriety so I had the chance to find it.

Three years later, I saw a notice about the first IRONMAN Florida, and I spontaneously signed up for it. **NO ONE** understood that choice. I'll never forget my dad's response—"You don't know how to swim." He was right, but in my gut, I knew it was the right choice for me and that I'd figure it out. Obviously, I was right.

In 2001, I made a spontaneous decision to start Racing for Recovery. The name "Racing for Recovery" just came to me, and I ran with it. I didn't say, "Wow, sounds cool, but let me think about it for another six weeks and see if I can come up with something else." I spent those six weeks building the next step of Racing for

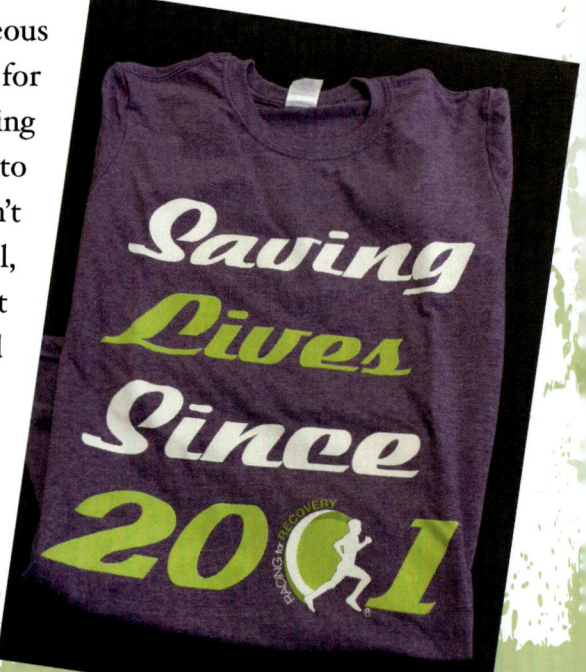

Recovery. When I walked through this building the first time, I mapped everything that I could do with it, every way we could grow, and I knew it was the one. I was thoroughly confused when someone asked where we were going to look next—why would I look anywhere else when this was it? I was already on to next steps, I needed to figure out how to get this building. Wandering around other buildings would have just distracted me from that.

Learning to trust myself and my intuition has been very important to my success. Some of the most critical moments in Racing for Recovery have been settled with these quick decisions that just felt right, that I didn't spend too much time questioning, very natural and easy. I've found that when you think things to death, you're not being responsible—you're doubting yourself, you're not trusting yourself. Allow yourself to be inspired 100%. I'm not sure if it was Albert Einstein, but someone smart once said, "I think 99 times and find nothing. I stop thinking, swim in silence and the truth comes to me." Once you've chosen sobriety, chosen healing, chosen to make the right decisions, you get to know yourself better. You learn to swim in that silence. You build your self-esteem and self-worth; you build a gut you can trust. It doesn't feel reckless to believe in your dreams, and the results are a lot more productive. At this point, when I question my gut intuition, that's when I make mistakes—that's usually when things don't work.

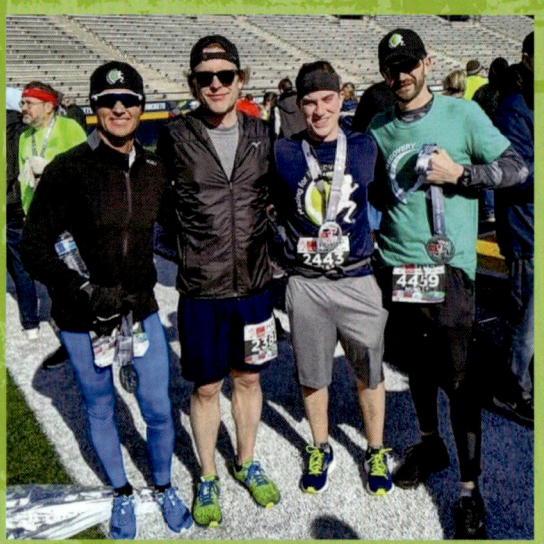

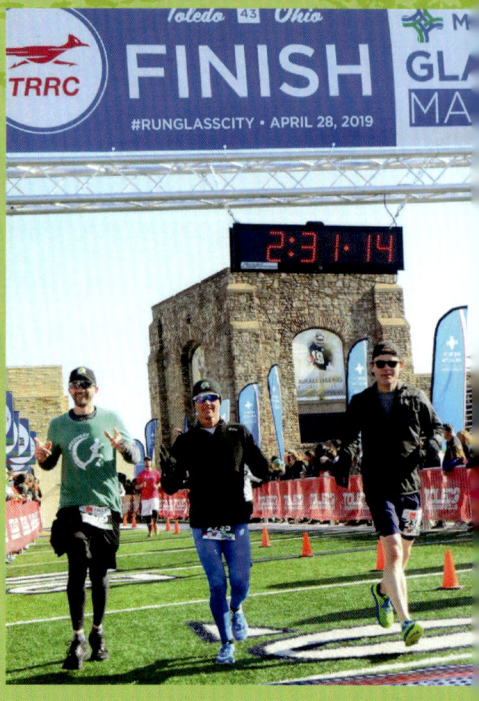

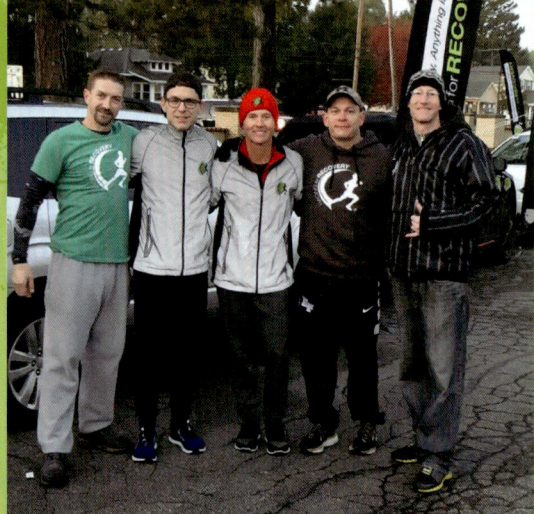

Using the benefits of exercise at the Glass City Half Marathon, Racing for Recovery 5k, and at IRONMAN Atlantic City 70.3

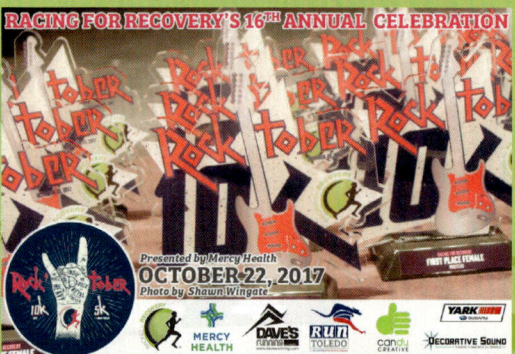

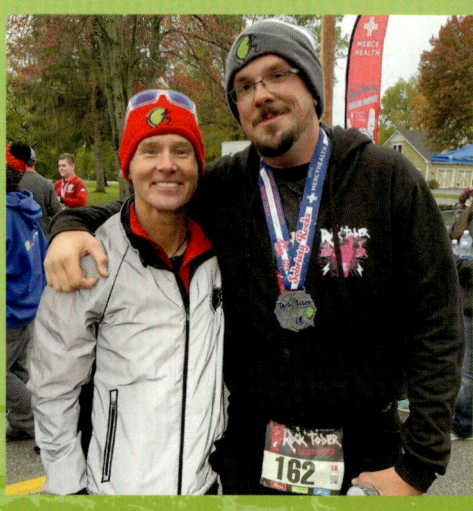

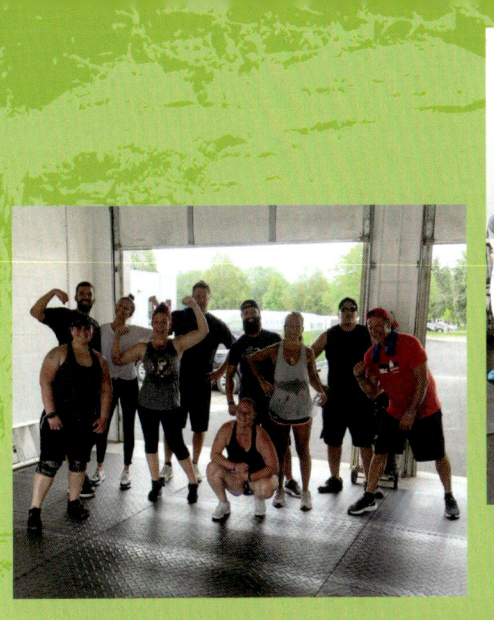

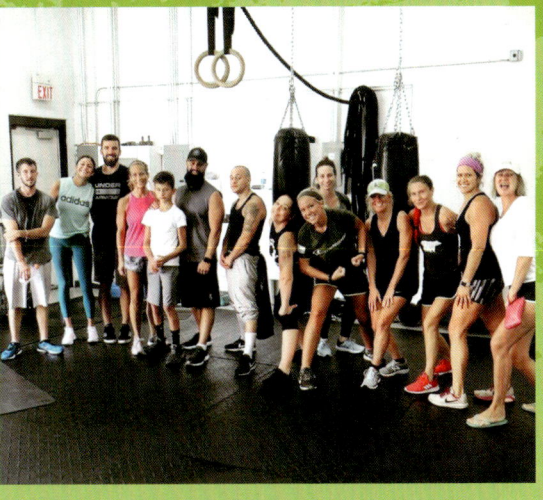

Racing for Recovery group
exercise sessions

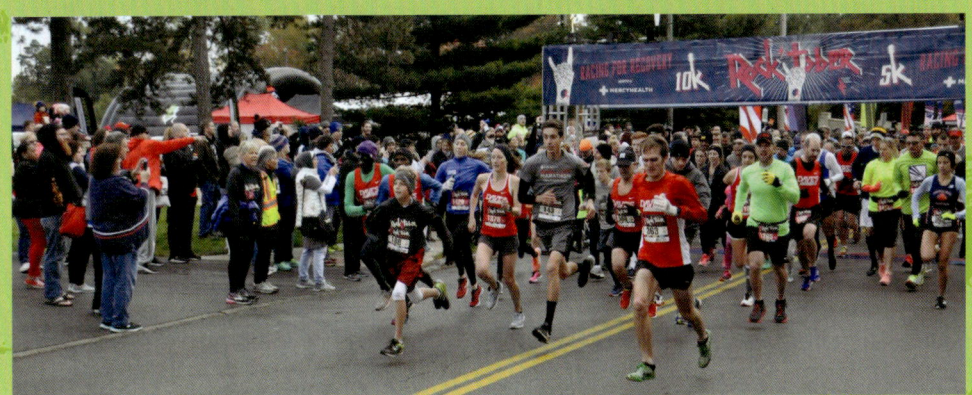

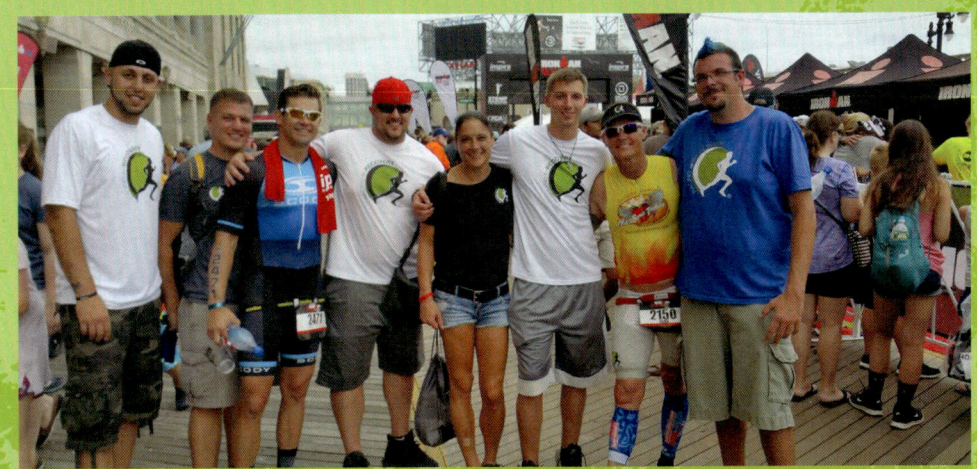

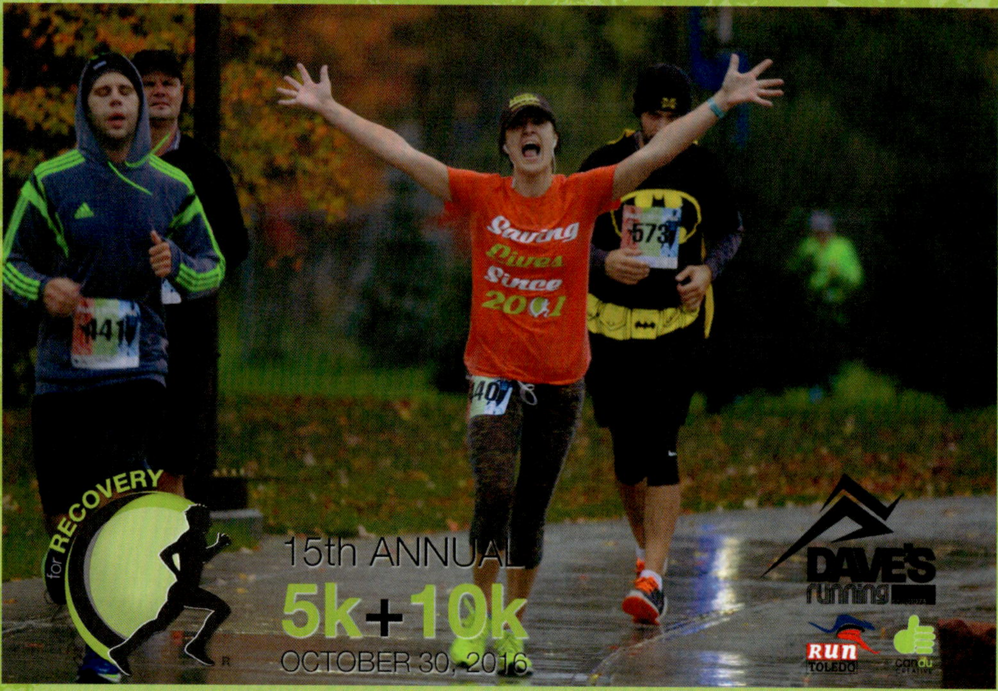

Saving Lives Since 2001
RECOVERY
15th ANNUAL
5k+10k
OCTOBER 30, 2016
DAVE'S running
RUN TOLEDO


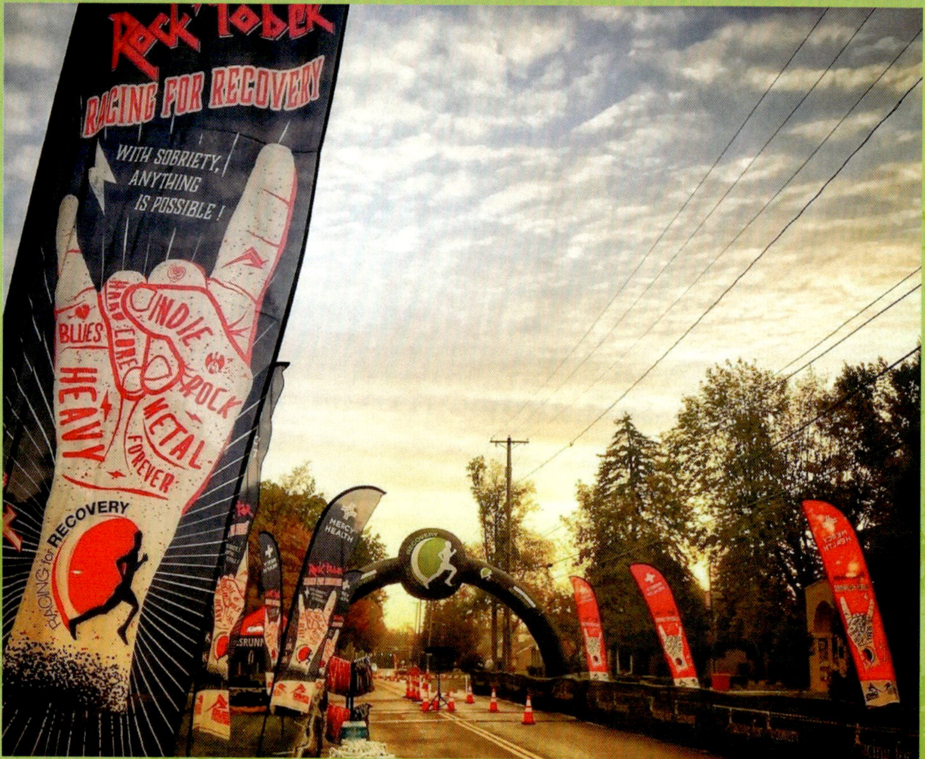

ROCK'TOBER
RACING FOR RECOVERY
WITH SOBRIETY, ANYTHING IS POSSIBLE!
INDIE
ROCK
METAL
FOREVER
BLUES
HEAVY
HARD CORE
RACING for RECOVERY

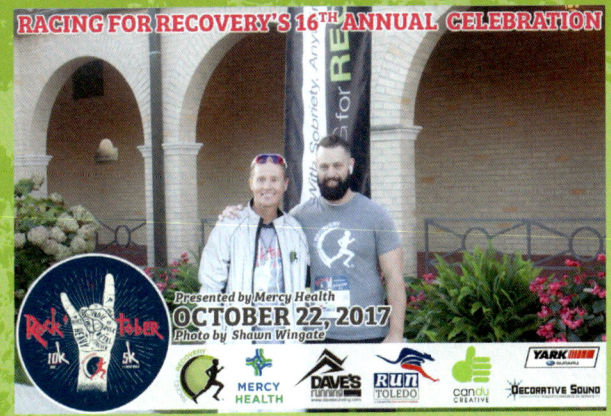

*Presented by Mercy Health*
**OCTOBER 22, 2017**
*Photo by Shawn Wingate*

My right hand man that allows me to fulfill my life's purpose
- Todd Bieber

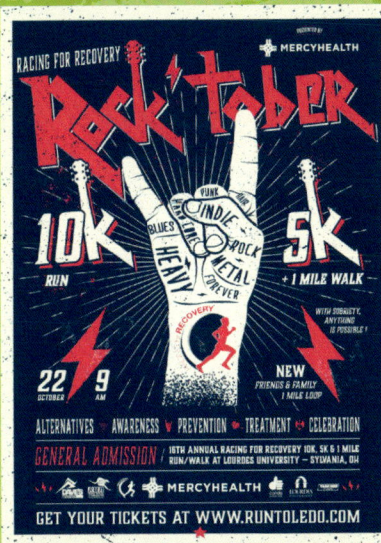

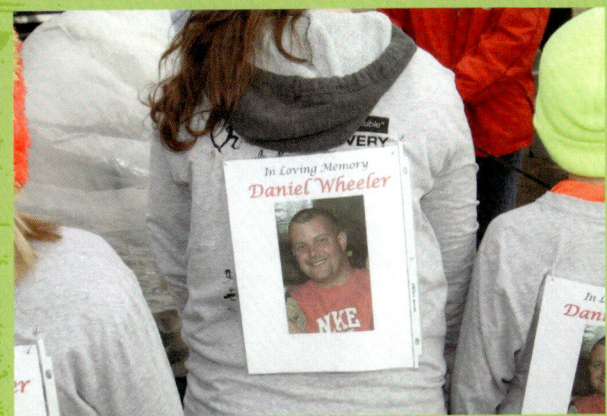

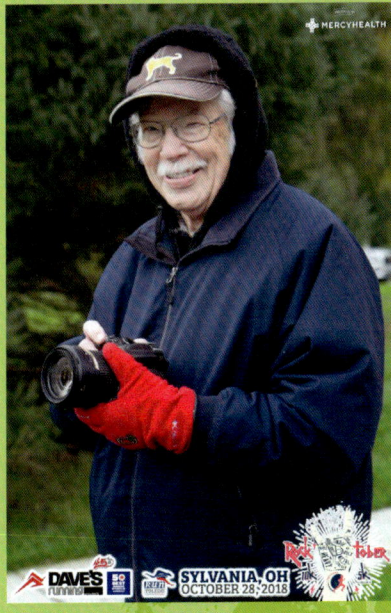

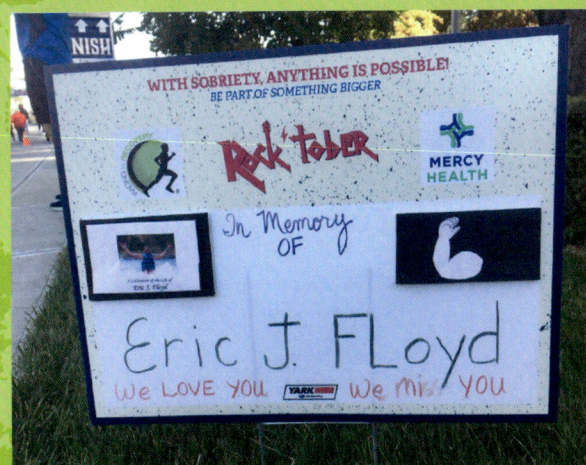

Pictures from our annual Racing for Recovery 5k

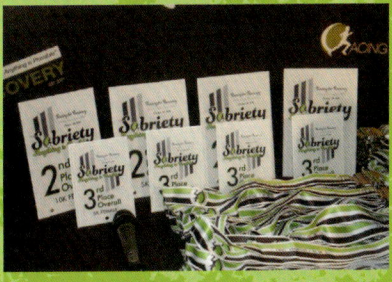

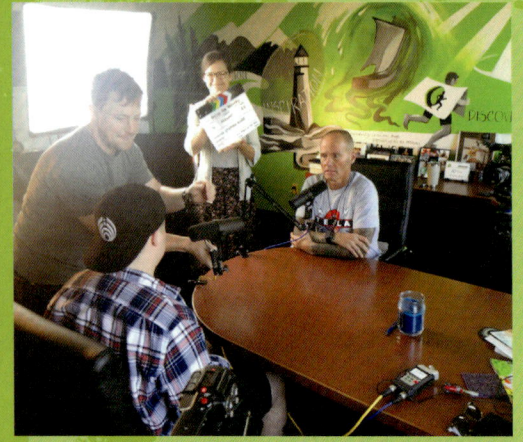

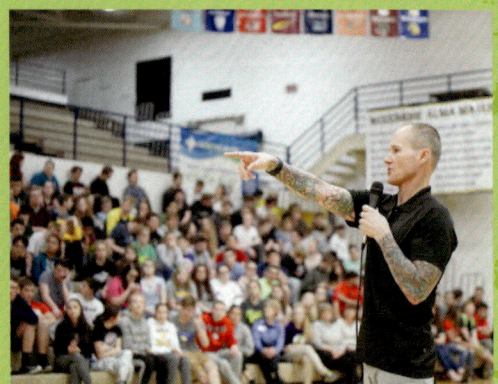

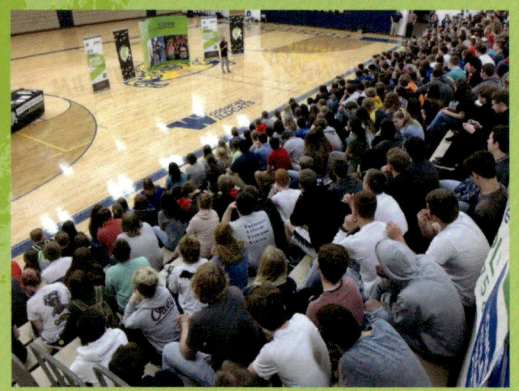

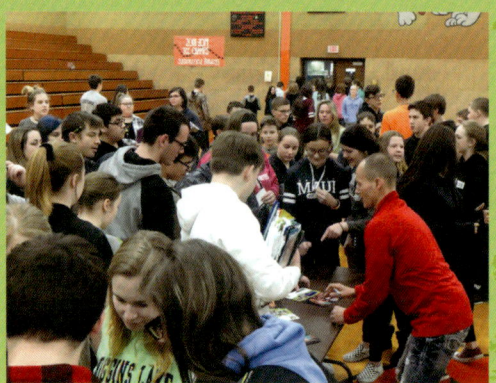

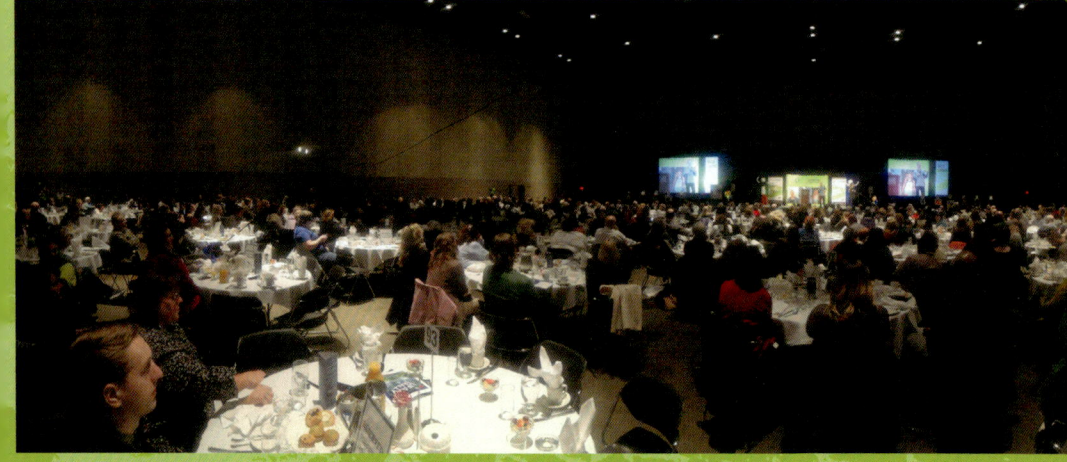

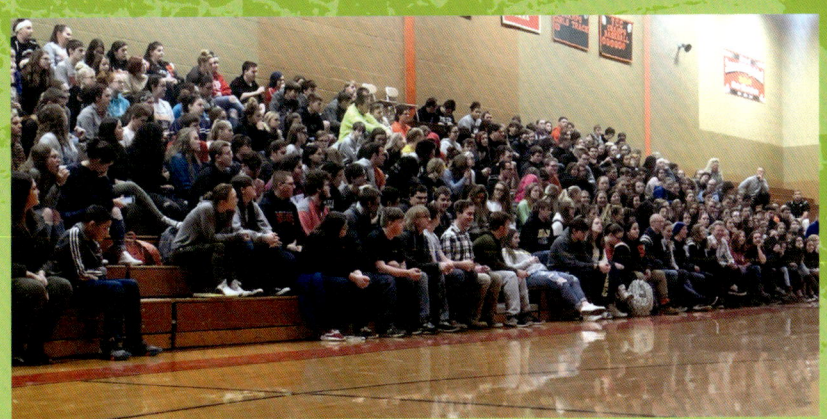

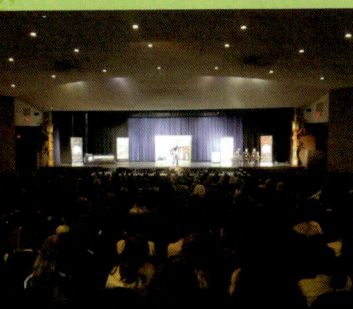

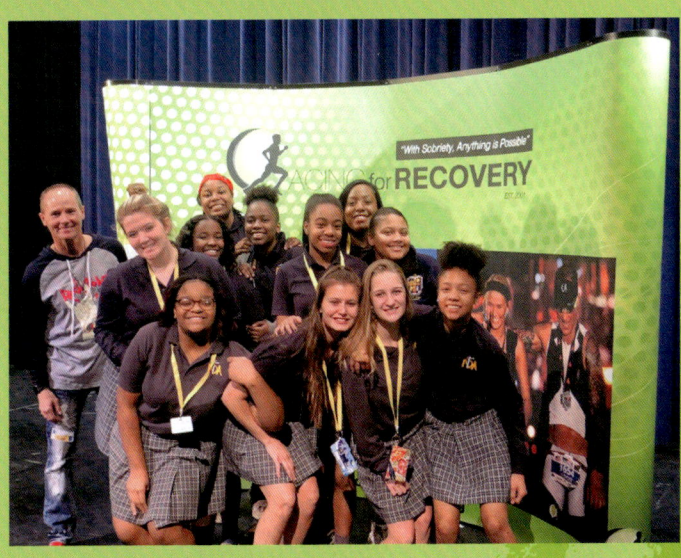

Speaking to junior high and high school students throughout Ohio and Kentucky and speaking to drug treatment agencies in Lansing, Michigan.

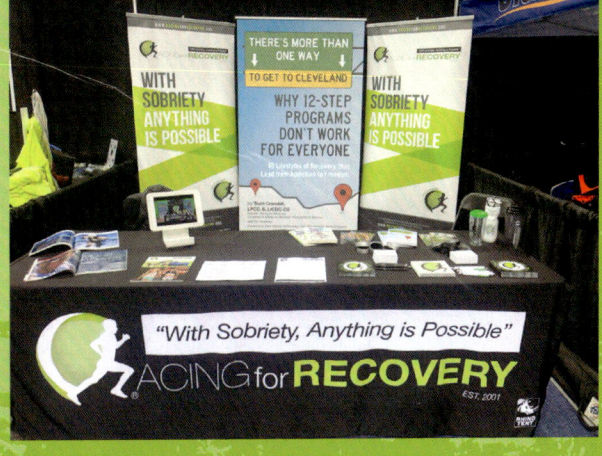

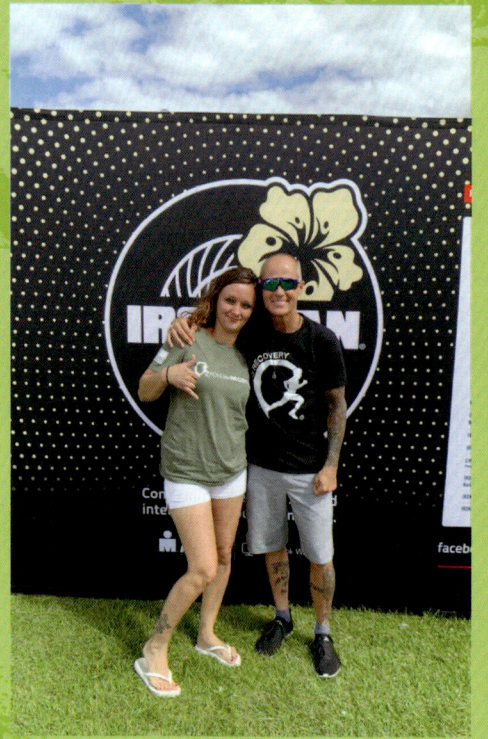

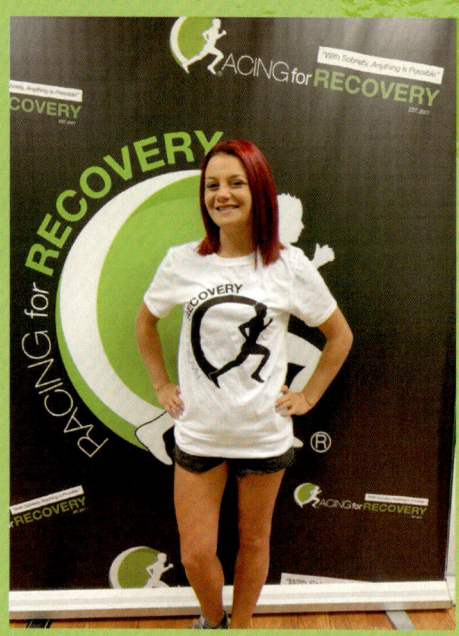

Below: Racing for Recovery Success Story
Megan Kelley. Sober Date 5-3-18

Above: Racing for Recovery Success Story
Faye Zerbe. Sober Date 11-27-18
IRONMAN Trevor City

IRONMAN Traverse City 70.3 2019

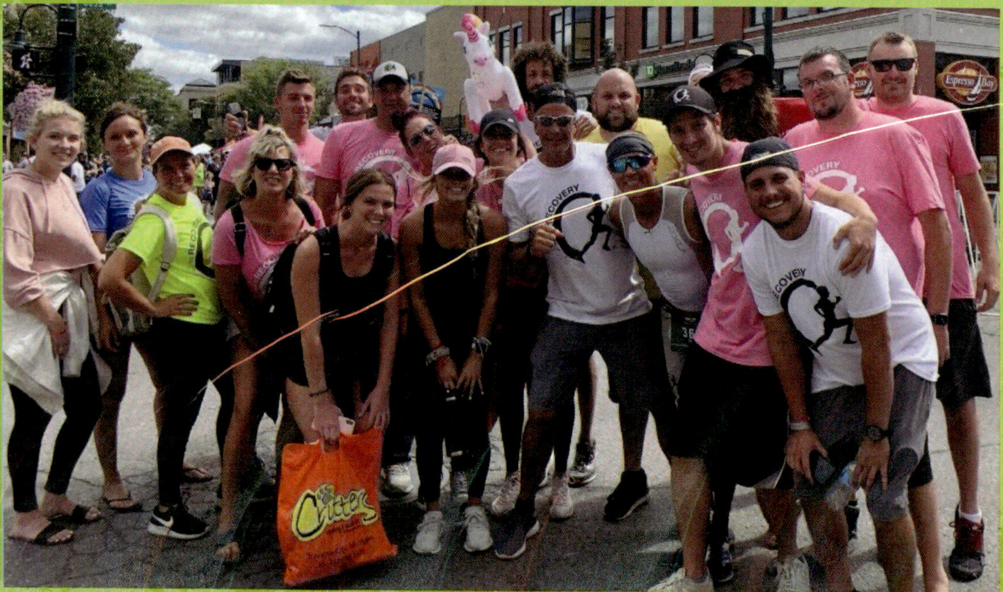

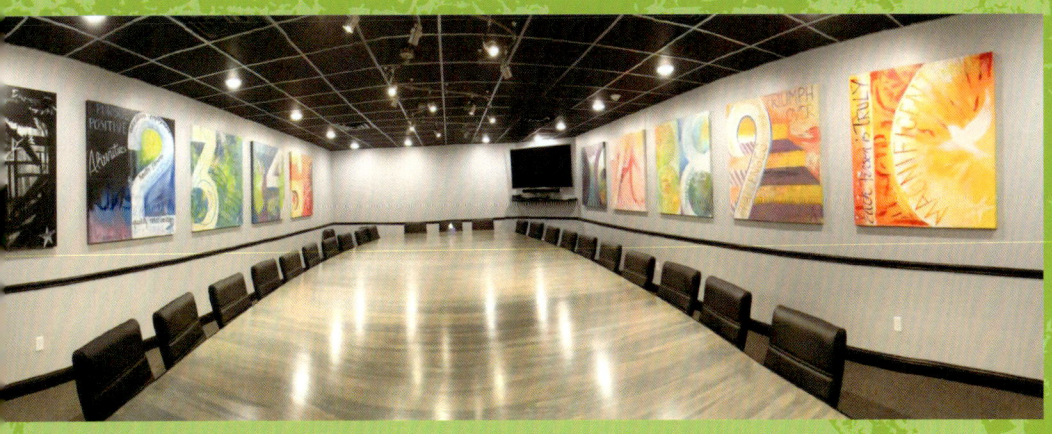

One of two Racing for Recovery education rooms

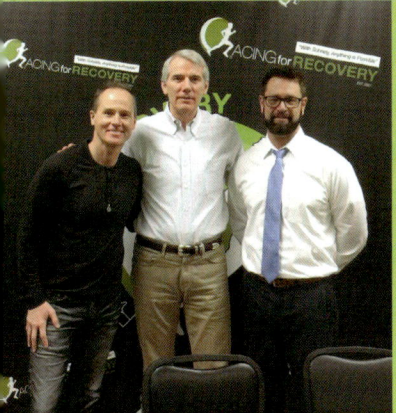

Left: With Senator Rob Portman and Racing for Recovery Executive Director Todd Bieber

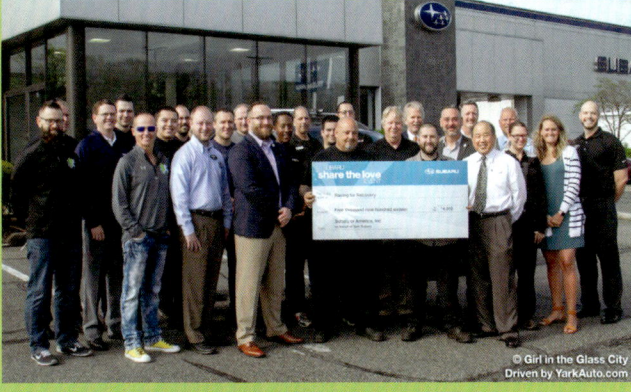

Receiving a kind donation from Yark Subaru

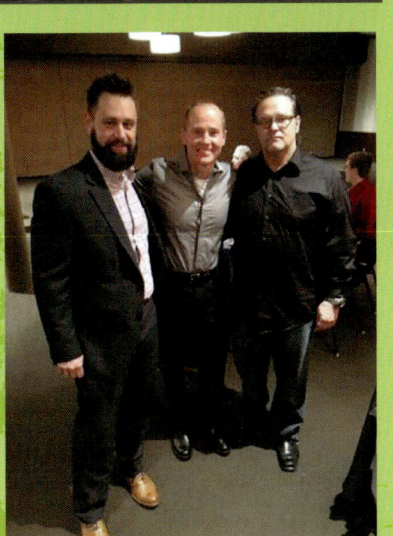

At the Jefferson Awards in Toledo, Ohio

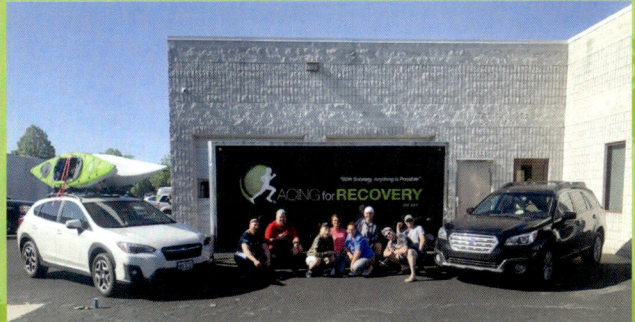

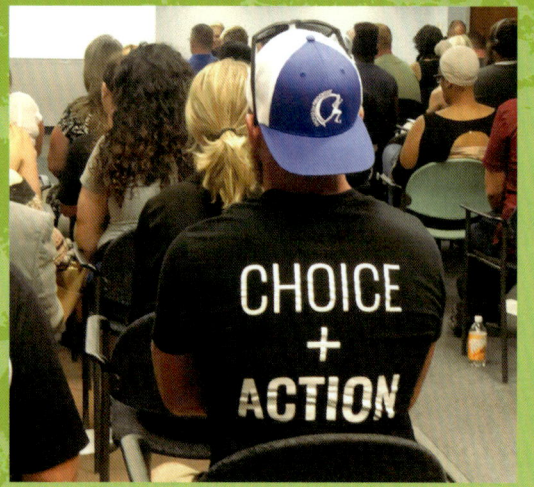

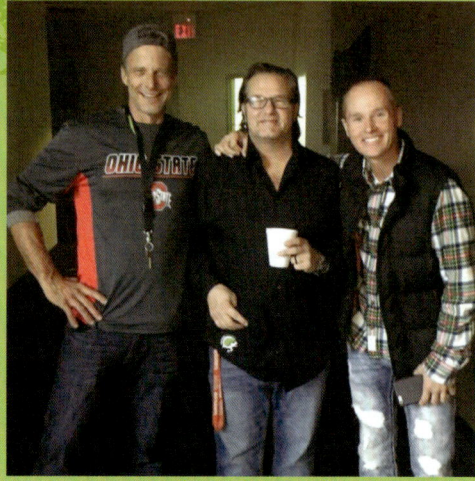

Great sober friends and staff Jeff and Dan

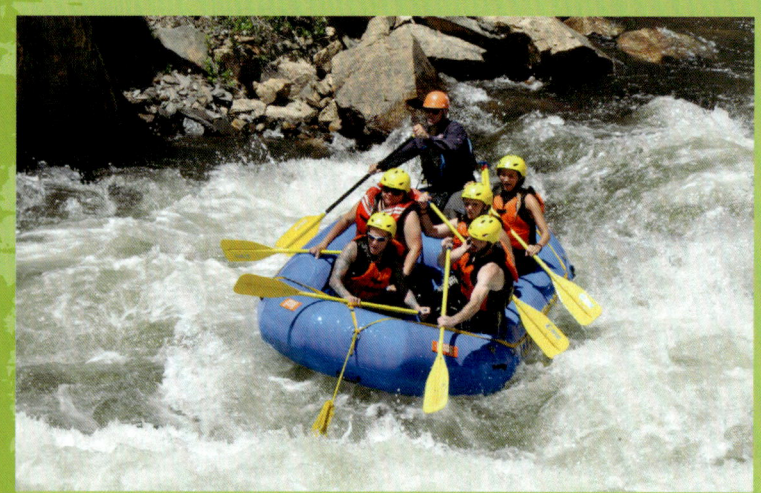

With Racing for
Recovery peers
whitewater
rafting
and enjoying
life the week
of IRONMAN
Boulder

Glass City Marathon Expo

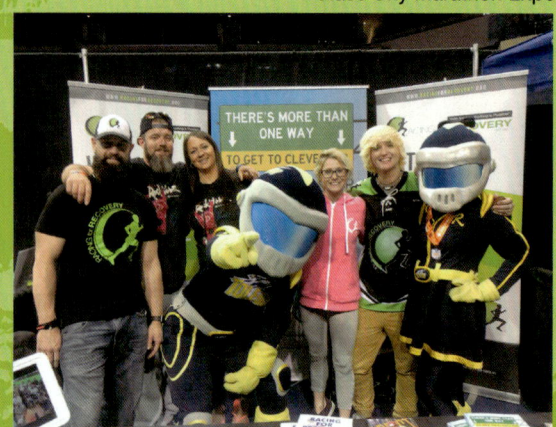

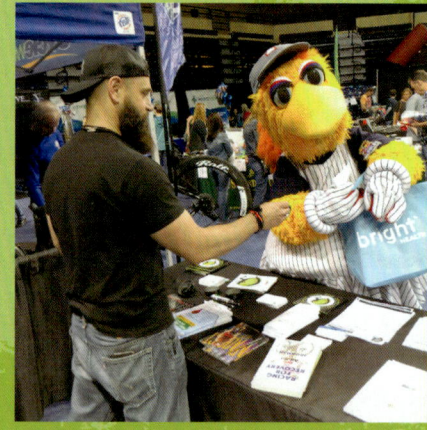

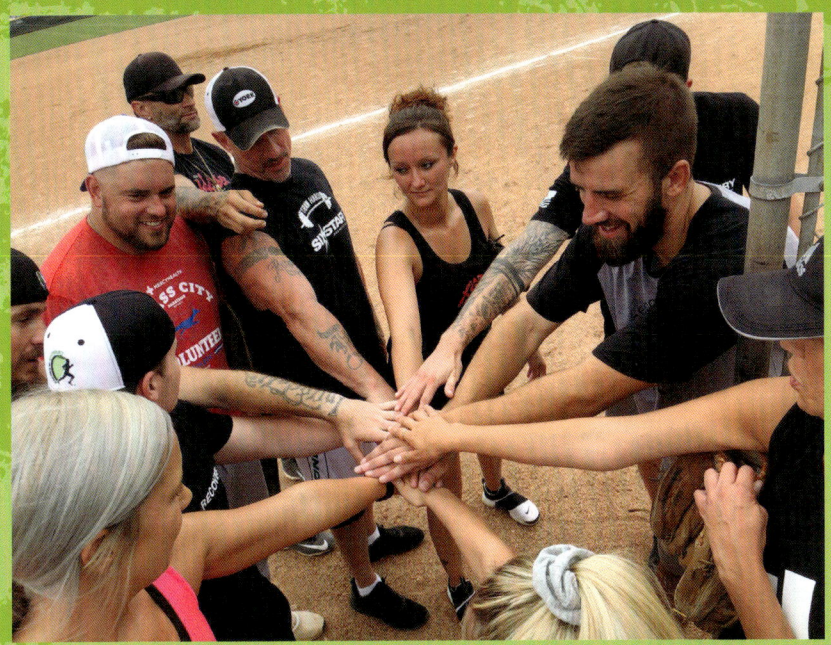

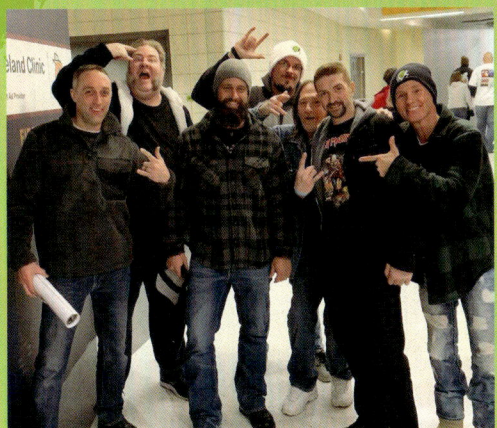

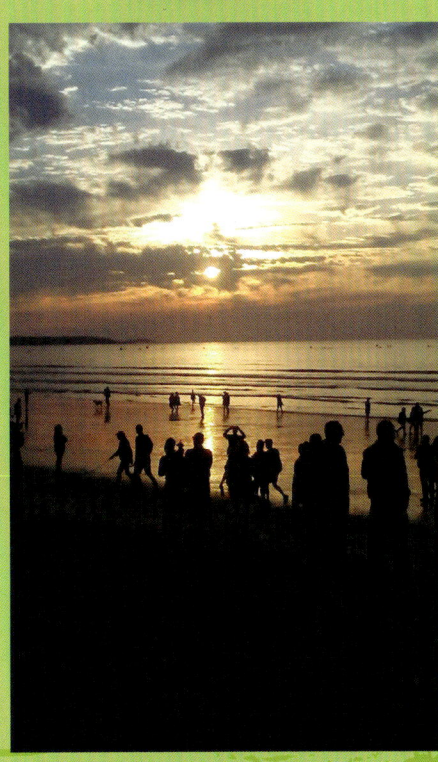

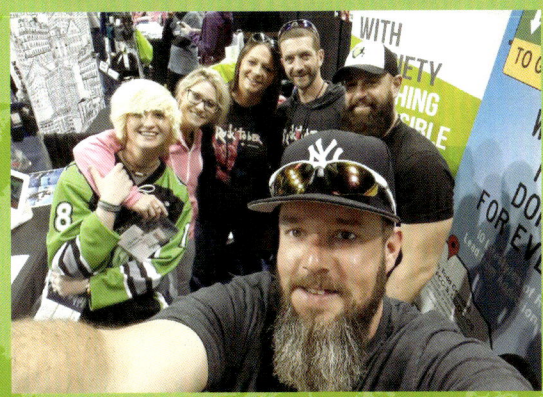

ABOVE: IRONMAN Maine 2018
Another great trip with Racing for Recovery
peers who are over a year sober now.

Choose to find your life's purpose through your passion, and keep a clear idea of what you are passionate about clear in your mind. If you're making decisions to support and pursue your passion and you keep it in balance with healing, sobriety, and love, you're going to choose right.

## WHAT IF I DON'T KNOW WHAT I'M PASSIONATE ABOUT?

With sobriety, anything is possible. Some things still take time to achieve, though. A lot of people come into my office thinking, "Hey man, I haven't used in three months, I want to start my own organization and be a counselor." It's my job to pump the brakes on some of that and channel it into more healing. We've got to walk before we can run—but then, we can run like IRONMEN!

It took me years of sobriety and healing to even get the idea that I had a purpose in life.

But I still chose passion.

I never would have found my life's purpose if I hadn't been trying new things, doing cool stuff that I was excited about. Sometimes we get stuck looking at what we don't want, who we don't want to become and what we don't like. It is valuable to pivot to exploring the positives—what we like, where we feel best and most alive, and who we are being when we are proud of our choices and the results we've created. You don't have to know everything you're passionate about and you don't have to know your life's purpose all in one sudden flash—finding out those things piece by piece, moving towards them, adding them to your life, are the greatest thrill of all.

It can take time for people in recovery to truly believe we deserve success and good things. Choosing passion and building that confidence is crucial to creating the balanced, holistic, healthy life you want and to grow in your sobriety. We feel better about ourselves and build self-worth and self-esteem when we engage in activities that we love. When you're doing what you like, there is less and less room in your life for self-destruction. You're never wasting time choosing to pursue your passions. All those experiences that you're building and skills you're acquiring are going to come in useful once you discover your life's purpose.

Choosing passion is recognizing that you can and should love yourself. You don't need to accomplish anything or become anything to deserve love. You have intrinsic value. When you

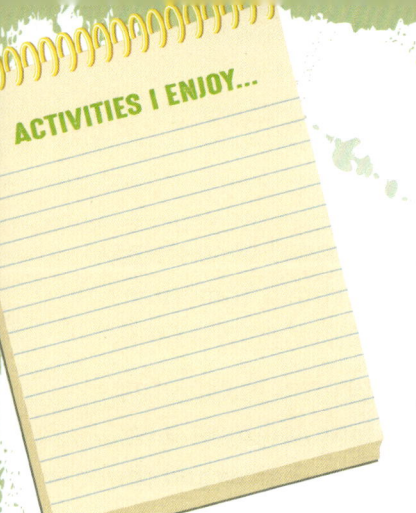

learn to love yourself, you realize at the same time you don't need to escape or numb your feelings. In fact, you feel good and want to feel life and everything that comes with it. Make a list of all of the activities you enjoy that promote sobriety. Pursue those activities. Make a list of those activities which make you feel vulnerable. Avoid those. Give yourself the time and space to explore who you are and what you love to do.

Take the time to appreciate the roles in your life that you never learned how to value as much as you should. We are all so much more than we give ourselves credit for, so much bigger and more important than we can see from inside our own heads. I'm still learning new things about myself every day, and learning to give myself credit. On the way to see Tesla the other night, my clients and I swung around and picked up my daughter Skylar from college nearby. We had an amazing time together, and when I dropped my daughter back off on our way home, one of my clients told me how cool it was to watch me be a dad. Not in Racing for Recovery mode or in counselor mode or in runner mode—all the things I do that I know people find inspiration in—but in being a dad, in loving my kids. It made me feel awesome, because it's one of the jobs I love best, and it's one of the hardest to quantify. There's a lot of "World's #1 Dad" mugs in the world, but you can't really compare your personal records. You hope you're doing a good job and just work on always getting better. It's important to pay attention to the things you're passionate about and grow your skills, even when you can't measure them.

Choosing passion is choosing gratitude, and that can be one of the mindset shifts that takes the most healing to develop. It took me many years to fully appreciate how incredible my life is. I was blind to my blessings, even my family, education, physical fitness, emotional wellness, friends, business, etc. I can now look at my life with appreciation. I understand that I have worked hard to get to where I am and through that hard work has come amazing support. I don't feel entitled to anything. I feel blessed and surrounded by grace, humility, and gratitude. When I accomplish life-long goals or small tasks, I constantly feel this sense of gratitude. It is a pillar of my sobriety and my work.

Now that I'm older, it's kind of weird to see what happened to many of the kids I grew up with who were "normal," who just coped with life. They graduated with good grades, finished up college in four years, got the job, got married, got the house, had kids, and boom, they settled into doing this for the next sixty years. I found that the route of self-destruction, if you choose to heal and then commit to fully live, makes you more appreciative of what life is really all about. Those of us who made worse decisions, who put ourselves through harder consequences, really value and treasure the benefits of our better choices. We fought harder and really understood how bad things could get, and we overcame it. We can't take the good things in our lives for granted, because they're miracles—miracles that we earned after we sometimes thought that we never could, and often thought we didn't deserve.

I am blessed to feel the joy of overcoming the obstacles and challenges that have beset my path to and through sobriety. I used to look back at my childhood despair and just feel angry—I didn't deserve that! I wouldn't wish the absolute despair I felt on anyone. It was crippling. I remember coming home drunk countless times, holing up in my room with my headphones and listening to music in the complete darkness. It still makes me incredibly sad to think about those times, but now it also makes me grateful. Melissa and I have four beautiful kids who, despite their genes, are emotionally healthy and have self-respect. They are so well-adjusted, kind, intelligent, empathetic, and caring. My sadness as a child formed the decisions I made about who I was going to be as a parent and what I valued. It taught me how to reach out and how to listen and when to seek help. My sadness became something beautiful because I was finally able to take lessons from it and use them to create something amazing.

**CHOOSING PASSION IS CHOOSING GRATITUDE AND CHOOSING TO FIND THE BEAUTY IN TRAGEDY.**

Those are nice words, Hallmark words. When you say something like that, everyone will agree and move on without thinking much about it.

Something we rarely talk about: Gratitude is shocking.

True gratitude scares people.

They don't have it, and they're upset when you have it.

People talk about being grateful for the good things in their lives, but until you are grateful for the worst things that ever happened to you, you're just enjoying nice things.

Ready for this?

My mother's suicide was the best thing that has ever happened to me.

I said this publicly at one of our support group meetings maybe five years ago, and some people really freaked out.

Am I happy my mom killed herself? Not at all.

Am I condoning suicide? Of course not.

My mom's suicide derailed me emotionally and led to my choices to use drugs. But the paths that I took to heal from my trauma has brought me every gift I have today. It has given me my life's purpose. I am grateful to have survived and I am blessed to have healed and embraced the opportunity that healing has afforded me to help others.

Trauma breaks you. Addiction keeps you broken. Healing and passion allow you to pick up those pieces and create something beautiful and special. When you are proud of who you are, the person you've made and the things you've done with all those pieces, you are grateful. When you've been cut on the sharpest edges of life and of yourself, you have a deeper understanding of how bad things can be. You have a deeper understanding of how good things can be. Your life is richer because of the worst thing that ever happened to you once you overcome it. You turned something that most people consider some sort of misery and death experience into something empowering.

Choose passion and your life's purpose will become clear. Embrace every part of yourself, even when it makes others frightened or angry. Don't hide and wait until you are perfect. You are valid, and every choice you make can help you grow into the person you are meant to be.

## WHAT IF I FAIL?

As a kid, failing even a small quiz can feel like the end of the world, let alone tests, classes, and grades. No adult moves past the possibility of failure either. I won't sugar coat it: anytime you're working towards anything, big or small, failure is a possibility.

Yes, I know—pointing out that failure looms around every corner might not sound like that trademark Racing for Recovery positivity, but I promise it is. I've spent the last twenty-five years facing challenges that often seemed impossible and triumphing, but that doesn't make me immune to failure. If anything, I've probably experienced more and bigger failures at a much closer range than a lot of people. I don't give myself anything to hide behind! I run straight towards my challenges, even when they look a lot like brick walls, and I've smashed face first into a few of them. I'll just give you three examples that should have been (according to any conventional wisdom) catastrophic, and the tools I had to develop to scoop my face back off the ground and keep moving.

## 1. FAILURES CAN BE ASSETS

When I was a kid, I almost always felt like I just didn't count. I just wasn't good enough at school, at church, or with my family. The one real exception was at the hockey rink—that was my home. Hockey was a lifeline for me when nothing else was. I knew in my heart that I was going to be a professional hockey player. I had my whole life planned out around it: I was going to move to Canada and get into the National Hockey League. I didn't need an education. Everything would be OK.

Don't get me wrong—I was a great hockey player, and hockey

was a good outlet for me when I was a kid. But I was trying to cover a big hole in myself with a tiny, puck-shaped Band-Aid, and by the time I was in high school, it just wasn't cutting it. I chose to cover over that hole with drugs and alcohol, and that choice cost me a hockey career. I failed, big time—failed myself, my coach, my team, and my dream.

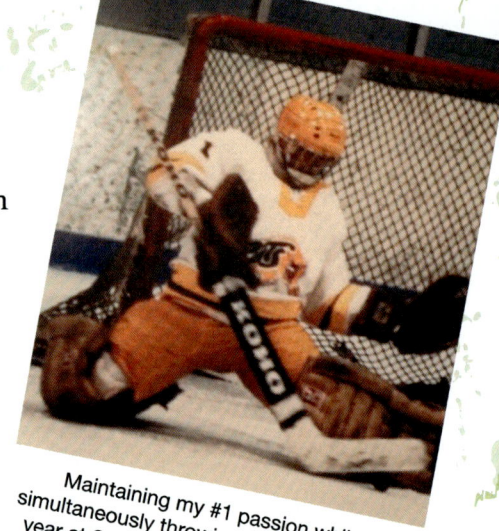

Maintaining my #1 passion while simultaneously throwing it away my junior year at Sylvania Northview High School

When my son started playing hockey, I took him up to an arena in Michigan for a game. Walking in, I had to point out a picture on the wall.

"Hey man, you're a big Montreal Canadiens fan—see this goalie? He used to watch me play from the bench—he was my backup."

He was impressed and pretty amazed, but we didn't talk much about it until the ride home, when he asked me if I wished I'd made it as a hockey player.

I looked at him and answered honestly: no. If I would have done that, right now I'd just be signing old hockey cards. I probably wouldn't have had my kids or my wife. I certainly wouldn't have had Racing for Recovery. I could have had a good life, but I don't know that I would have had a great one. I have everything in my life now that I ever wanted.

Abandoning my hockey dreams was probably the second biggest trauma in my life after my mom's suicide, but those two things were the catalysts for every choice I've made since. I took those traumas and made them into assets. I found my life's purpose in them and built a fulfilling life helping people. Everything I am today was built on those choices, and I'm really, really proud of who I am and what I've built.

Don't choose to fail. (If my last choice had been drugs over hockey, I absolutely would not have this amazing life. I had to make many, many better choices to get here.) But when you do fail, don't despair. Turn those failures into assets by learning from them and growing and making better choices. As long as you're alive, your world has literally countless possibilities for success beyond your wildest dreams.

## 2. DON'T ASSUME YOU'LL FAIL BEFORE YOU TRY

Even though I never became a professional hockey player, if I hadn't ever been seriously involved with hockey, I wouldn't be sitting here today—literally, I wouldn't be sitting in my office. Six months after Racing for Recovery moved into our incredible facilities, the owner of the building realized she needed to sell it. I needed a million dollars, immediately, or I was going to lose everything, and my bank account was a little more than a little short. I went to the most competent, most capable person I knew, the man most likely to be able to do the impossible—my former hockey coach, Coop.

Jim Cooper carried me into the hockey rink for the first time when I was five years old, and no matter how many times he watched me make bad choices and face gnarly consequences, he's always been there for me. He believed in me before I believed in myself, and when I started to get an inkling that there was something good—something really great, actually—inside of me.

He even financed my first book. There's a big difference between a book printing and a million-dollar question, though, so I didn't know what to expect when I told him about my situation. I knew I only had two possible choices, though—to ask for help or to give it all up. As someone who spends all day everyday counseling people to ask for help when they need it, I couldn't just back down now.

RACING
FOR
RECOVERY

From
Addict
to
IRONMAN

TODD CRANDELL

JOHN HANC

Don't let the possibility of almost-certain failure keep you from choosing to pursue big dreams. Ask for help when you need it, even when it seems like an impossibly big favor. I am overcome with gratitude and humility every day, stepping into this building that Coop helped us acquire, so that we can continue helping the thousands of people who come to us.

## 3. NOT ALL FAILURES ARE PERMANENT

When I realized Racing for Recovery was my life's purpose, I knew I was up against some steep challenges. To do everything I was dreaming about, I needed to become a licensed professional clinical counselor with supervisor status (LPCC-S). Without that credential, I wouldn't be qualified to provide clinical services in my own office or to supervise any of my counselors...

And that meant I would have to go back to school.

That was hard. I wasn't a good student when I was a kid; even though I'd gained way more self-confidence by the time I chose to start up again as an adult, it still wobbled in the classroom. I was lucky to have some incredible professors, who taught me as much about myself and my capabilities as they did about the subject matter. (Huge shout out to all the educators who put in the extra effort to help their students thrive—you make all the difference in our lives!) I will always be especially grateful for Professor Barbara Masten, who I was lucky enough to work with while completing my undergraduate degree at Lourdes

University. I'd always rushed through my work, making mistakes and truly believing those mistakes defined me. Her classroom structure helped me relax and not hurry my work. The two most important lessons she taught me weren't on the syllabus, but I carried them close to me through all my other classes: **1) I COULD DO IT, AND 2) THERE WERE GOOD PEOPLE WHO WOULD HELP.**

Finishing my coursework was only the first hurdle, though. The LPCC exam loomed over me, and it made me feel sick just thinking about it. I'd been convinced for a long time that some people have a gift for taking tests; others could study hard and be successful; and then, there was a third group, my group, of people who were born to bomb.

But I powered through...

And failed.

And failed.

And failed again.

Once, I was only two points away from a passing grade. Another time, I was just one point shy.

It could have been devastating (it definitely wasn't easy). I might have even quit if I didn't have a secret weapon: Alyson M. Carr, PhD, LMHC.

Alyson Skyped with me for weekly tutoring session and helped me get my mind right for the exam. She helped me understand that the way I thought about counseling was different than the type of thinking I needed to do to pass the test. I had to learn what it took to qualify to do my work, not to simply do my work. It was tough to swallow, but her words stuck with me: "Todd, you do this profession with heart and passion, which is awesome, but you have to learn how to think like the exam so you can pass it, so you can utilize your heart and passion for the clients you work with."

Earning my LPCC is one of my proudest accomplishments. I worked for four years and took the exam six times before I passed. (Yeah, of course I cried actual tears of joy!) Many might be discouraged or embarrassed by this, but I feel like it is a badge of honor. I kept working and trying; I earned my credentials.

DON'T GIVE UP

Some things in life you only get one shot at, but more often than not, failing something isn't the end of that road unless you choose to turn off. Many people would have given up on the LPCC exam after their first, third, or fifth failed attempts. My dream was so much bigger, and walking away from this one test would have meant walking away from my life's purpose. Failing before you succeed at something hard can help you understand how truly valuable it is.

I choose to pursue a lot of big dreams, so I face a lot of big failures. The idea of facing catastrophic failure is enough to keep a lot of people from trying. Of course, the idea of failing bugs me too—that's why I completely throw myself into everything I choose to do. Whether I succeed or fail, I know I've left it all on the field. I commit to my progress and I commit to myself. We all get discouraged sometimes, but we can't confuse a need to rest with a need to quit. We might have to change our courses or our tactics, but it's crucial to keep our major goals in mind at all times.

There is one failure a lot of people accept as inevitable that I just don't accept: the idea that relapse is part of recovery. Some people that come into Racing for Recovery are completely blown away when I share a simple truth that I know from personal experience: **YOU NEVER HAVE TO DRINK OR USE DRUGS AGAIN.**

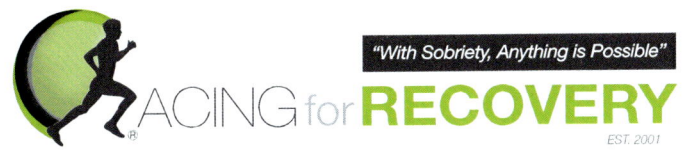

"With Sobriety, Anything is Possible"
RACING for RECOVERY
EST. 2001

# CHOOSE LOVE

When we are hurting, we hurt the people around us. We isolate ourselves, alienate ourselves, and act badly towards the people in our lives. Pain draws us inwards and becomes our only focus, making us selfish and self-centered. A major part of healing and living an awesome life is connecting with other people—loving and being loved. We are social animals, and we are only happy with strong connections to other people; that's what makes life good. Learning how to treat the people in our lives and how to build and rebuild healthy relationships is important.

## WHAT IF CHOOSING THE RIGHT THINGS ISOLATES ME FROM MY FRIENDS?

Kids often came to my house for sleepovers or to play hockey in my driveway or skate on the nearby pond. Or they'd come out to my grandma's house, where I spent nearly every weekend. Honestly, I liked that better—her house was welcoming. I felt out of place everywhere but my grandma's and on the ice. Those were my secure spots, where I felt good enough. I felt disconnected from my dad, stepmom, and brother. I felt like the bad, broken kid, the one who didn't belong.

[I've actually always looked up to my brother, even though he's eight years younger than me. He was a great kid—never got into drugs (seeing the mess I was helped), went to Catholic high school and then a good college. Now, he's got a beautiful family and he's a world-famous yoga instructor. My dad makes comments now like "My two sons both take care of themselves by doing what they want to do," which makes me feel amazing—proud of myself, proud of my brother, and proud of my parents. It's nice to finally be one of the good kids!]

I had a naturally effusive personality. I was enthusiastic about playing, and my enthusiasm was infectious. I enjoyed creating a Hey, this is going to be awesome! tone, and my spirited and positive attitude attracted the other kids.

I've carried this trait into my adult life. It is evident, and probably essential, in my organization. Often, I have a vision, and the vision inspires me to act. By acting with inspiration and enthusiasm, people are also inspired and buy into the vision.

One of my first visions was for a bike race—a **BIG EVENT.**

Success.

Because of its popularity, it evolved into a weekly activity we called canning. This involved us racing through the neighborhood on trash day and kicking over the garbage cans (sometimes before the garbage truck had arrived—we should have probably taken more responsibility for the trash that sometimes spilled).

What became clear was that I could organize people to do cool things when I was enthusiastic about it.

Remember, your energy is contagious. Because of this, it is important to choose your energy well. If you're enthusiastic, others will be too.

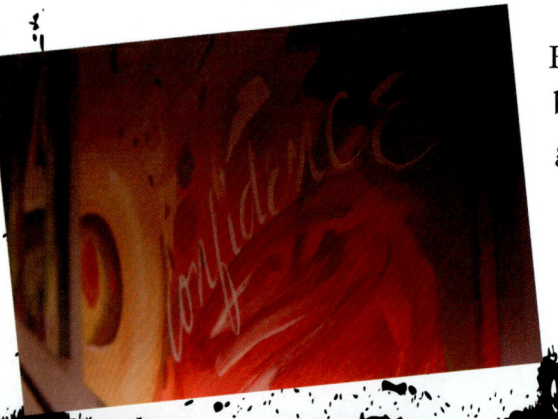

By gaining the confidence to believe in yourself and your good choices, you are able to choose love by making it easier for your friends to choose the right things alongside you. You become a leader, and your choices impact more and more lives in a positive way.

The kids who took part in my bike races would have said I was a leader, but anyone who saw me in a classroom sure wouldn't have! Being asked a question in school made me physically uncomfortable—like, want-to-crawl-out-of-my-own-skin levels. Ironically, when someone else answered the question correctly, it would only decrease my self-confidence: Hey, I knew that. I should have raised my hand. My confidence and self-esteem were conditional.

When we value ourselves, we have self-esteem. When we have self-esteem, we do not do things to hurt ourselves. We make choices to improve ourselves, like being active in school, church, sports, and our communities. Being active in these organizations cultivates our self-esteem, while simultaneously developing our leadership skills.

When you commit to making the right choices, it means you can't be a follower. Choosing not to choose makes us vulnerable to leaders who don't have our best interests at heart, and we forfeit our power to make our own, best decisions. You might not be a leader all the time—no one is! If I'm on an airplane, I want the pilot

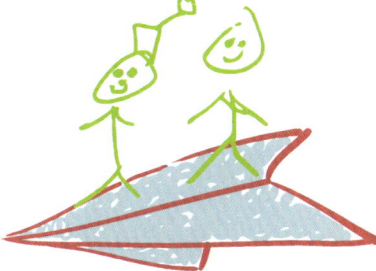

to fly it, because I have no expertise in flying. But I've still got to be the one who chooses where I'm going, even when I need someone else's help getting me there.

It's important to choose love when we're looking to other people for expertise to inform the choices we have to make. Sometimes we need people to lean on. We have questions. We can be confused or uncomfortable with life. It is important that we have people we trust in our lives. It's normal to be attracted to confidence in someone else, but when those people are really bullies or projecting confidence as a defense mechanism, they won't be satisfied to let you make your own decisions. Whether you're asking for guidance making a decision from a family member, friend, or authority figure, the choice is up to you, and the consequences will be yours to face.

Not everyone will be ready to make good choices, even among your closest friends. You might lose touch with some people you are very close to for a period of time, or even forever. Their decisions can't impact yours.

Some of those friends you think you've lost forever, though, will surprise you. Remember my buddy Dan? You met him walking into this book. He works the front desk here at Racing for Recovery.

I've known Dan since I was twelve. We were two of the best

hockey players to ever come out of Toledo, Ohio. He's also a miraculously smart dude (like, he somehow got me through Algebra 2 in high school, an Evel Knievel-esque stunt).

I did my first line of cocaine with Dan in the Sylvania Northview High School parking lot the first Friday of our senior year. I remember saying something to the effect of, "Wow, what a year this is going to be." And I was right—within four months, we'd snorted the opportunity to win Northview its first state title in hockey up our noses, gotten expelled, and ruined our chances at professional hockey careers.

About six months into my sobriety, I ran into Dan, who was still deeply struggling with addiction. He pleaded with me: "I can't live this way anymore. I need some help and a place to stay."

My grandma was an incredible person, a woman who was able to navigate the near-impossible twists and turns of supporting and loving a person struggling with addiction. She'd been kind enough to allow me to live with her while I was in recovery; then, she opened her home to Dan as well. We spent many days and nights laughing, listening to AC/DC, and going to support groups—healing. Dan and I were in each other's weddings and took our joint fantastic honeymoon together in Negril, Jamaica. I remember sitting on the beach, looking out into the beautiful blue ocean water and thinking, This is one true benefit of sustaining sobriety.

When Racing for Recovery secured our facility in the fall of 2016, Dan came back to simply volunteer. He learned the ins and out of the business side, came up with new 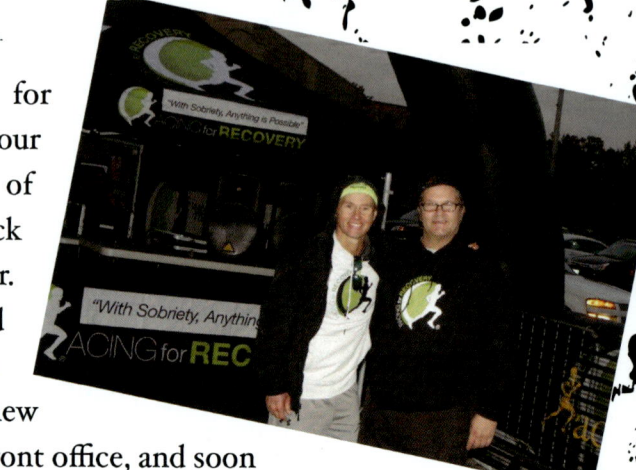 ways to improve our front office, and soon made himself and his amazing brain completely invaluable. Now, we both get to spend our days reaching out and helping people lead themselves out of addiction struggles.

Being a leader starts with leading yourself, whether or not anyone else is going to follow you, but you never know who is watching you and how you'll be able to help them as you build your own strength. When we walk confidently down our path and show others the great results, we naturally lead by example. People are often willing to follow good examples. You will not be alone for long, because there are other people who are just as sick of feeling sick as you were, people who were just waiting for someone to show them a better way to live.

## WHY ISN'T SEX MAKING ME FEEL BETTER?

I had my first kiss the summer before sixth grade. Well, sort of. One moment, we were just sitting in a tent; then she had her tongue in my mouth. I wasn't quite sure what was happening. I felt weird, like I had done something wrong. My curiosity escalated in pretty normal ways through junior high school. I knew I wanted to fool around, and poorly-lit basement parties provided opportunities to pair off and experiment.

Girls were always "more than just friends." I was interested in them. I was attracted to them, drawn to them. I wanted them to be the solution to my problems, to heal me, make me feel loved and not alone.

In high school, I started dating a very pretty, nice girl. We were a disaster together. We bonded over our emotional issues, and we were co-dependent on each other. When it was good, it was great, but when it was bad, it was devastating and sad.

Her father had left when she was two; her mom was great, but she worked a lot. It was fun to take advantage of her empty house after school, but driving home at night, it hurt me to know that she was alone. I cared about her.

The hard truth is that caring about someone doesn't heal you.

Loving people is great and important, but if you're a mess, people aren't Band-Aids. I was a mess. I was angry all the time, and we argued a lot. Yelling, smashed telephones, radios, and cassette tapes—I even broke a window on Good Friday, attempting to kick her stereo through it. Replacing glass is expensive; watching yourself emotionally tear down a person you love is worse.

I was seventeen the first time we had sex (January 1, 1984—the day that Van Halen released their album 1984). She had more experience, so she led the way. It felt like a milestone and an achievement in my life, but like that first kiss, I walked away feeling like I'd done something wrong.

Choosing to have sex can lead to many serious physical consequences, including pregnancy and STDs. I knew that. But I hadn't realized how emotionally loaded it could be. I was confused whether it was love, whether I knew what love was, whether I had to do it, whether I was supposed to do it, whether I wanted to keep doing it. It joined the pile of other choices I was making that weren't right for me. It made me feel more guilty and lowered my (already dangerously low) self-esteem.

Rather than facing this choice and dealing with my trauma, I chose to mask over it with more drugs, more alcohol, and more sex. We had sex with each other pretty much daily for the next two years. I also had sex with as many other women as possible, a rampage that continued for years after we'd broken up.

I never lied to the women I had sex with about being exclusive, but that didn't make me a good person. I was using them. No healthy, happy person goes out to just try and collect as many sexual partners as possible. I didn't have the "hunt" or "conquest" mentality (not to say this is a healthy approach to sexuality either—it isn't). I wanted them to heal me. I had to bond with every woman on a sexual level in order to feel a connection. I hated myself so much that I couldn't believe anyone else liked me without that "proof." I couldn't find anything good in myself, so I looked to other people, hoping they would show me where it was. When a woman would have sex with me, I took that as a sign she saw something good in me emotionally, that I had value. The more women that had sex with me, the more women agreed that I was worthwhile.

My self-esteem was so low that I couldn't even take that external validation at face value. It was puzzling to me that so many women would come to my dingy apartment and have sex with me, in my condition. I'd wonder aloud what was wrong with them, what was wrong in their lives, that they were willing to do this, that they thought it was a remotely good idea. The fact that they would have sex with me devalued them, in my eyes. It meant they had a problem.

How messed up is that?!? Pick up a girl to have sex with me in the hopes that her validation would heal me, fully convinced that any girl that would have sex with me is defective, so her validation isn't worth as much. I'd rigged the game. No one could win, not even me.

Messed up, yeah, but not uncommon. That's pretty much the name of the game for anyone who tries to use people for external validation.

I continued using women this way through my first year and a half of sobriety—even after I met Melissa. I remember meeting my wife for the first time and thinking, this is the girl for me. Initially, it was because of her looks, but very quickly, it was way more. It was her innocence and kindness, intelligence and emotional stability—and it didn't hurt that she wasn't struggling with addiction. This wasn't merely attractive, it was essential. I didn't have the foundation to be sober for two.

I do not know where I found the courage to ask her out on a date, but I did. She, however, refused to take part in the sexual mess I had going on: "Why would I get with you if you're doing that?"

My response? "Well, if you tell me that we're gonna be a thing, I'll quit doing this. If we're not gonna be a thing, then I'm gonna keep doing this."

I know, that's twisted. I had been having sex for a decade, but I'd never been in a healthy sexual relationship, because I'd never been healthy. I'd connected with Melissa in sobriety on a deep emotional level, but I had no experience with sex that wasn't, on a validation level, transactional.

Along with the potential physical consequences, sex is complicated and emotional. For people who struggle with emotional trauma, low self-esteem, and addiction, examining our choices around sex is important to healing and building healthy holistic lives. Millions of people in the United States, many of whom struggle with addictions, have been traumatized by sexual abuse. This can make engaging with sex in a healthy way even more complicated.

Understanding intellectually and emotionally why you are choosing to have sex is an example of being self-aware and self-confident. It's important for you to value your emotional and physical health and consider how they could be impacted by your sexual activities. Sex, like drugs, can't heal your emotional trauma. Using sex for external validation of your worth isn't a substitute for building your self-esteem.

Trauma and addiction alienate us from other people. They make it difficult to establish healthy connections. They make us selfish and self-centered—not because we're "bad people," but because we don't know who we can trust or how we can heal. Pain draws us inside our own heads. It's a loud alarm bell that makes it hard to really hear anything or engage with anyone in a meaningful way.

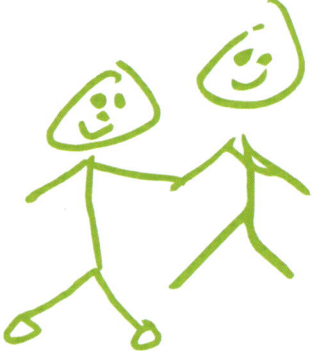

Choosing love is about learning how to connect with people in a meaningful way, whether that involves sex or not, learning to trust and how to empathize. It's about getting out of your own head and building the relationships that will make your life more joyful and meaningful. Choosing love is when you engage with people to enhance your life and theirs.

Choosing love means recognizing that healthy, fulfilling sex shouldn't seem like an obligation. It means not pressuring, coercing, manipulating, or forcing someone to engage with you sexually. It means not pressuring yourself into performing sexually when you cannot engage with it joyfully.

There are no sexual deadlines you have to hit—not for your first time and not in a relationship. It doesn't matter if your ninetieth birthday is looming or if you've gone on a million dates with someone—you're not a loser for waiting until you're ready. Having sex with someone once, twice, or two hundred times doesn't mean that you need to have more sex with them. There's no such thing as unreasonable boundaries, and there's no "point of no return" in healthy, consensual sex. Consent means more than "no means no"—it's an honest, joyful, and enthusiastic "yes!"

every step of the way. You're awesome, and you deserve that, and so does anyone cool enough to have sex with you.

## WHY DON'T PEOPLE TRUST ME?

I rarely get angry with Racing for Recovery clients, but I made an exception recently.

A woman stood up in our support group meeting and spoke about how she was sober and how great everything was. As she was talking, though, Dan showed me her court-ordered drug screen from earlier in the week. It was positive for cocaine.

We called her in next morning and I asked her to explain the results. It took quite a few rounds for her to finally admit she'd been using.

Now, I'm not naïve. People in the midst of addiction frequently spend a lot of time and energy hiding their choices. I wasn't immune—I hid my use and lied to my dad when I started to abuse drugs and alcohol. I don't begrudge my clients who are lying to me or lying to themselves about their drug use. I train almost every day with Andy, and when he decided he wanted to try a triathlon, Racing for Recovery made sure he had all the gear—the bike, the shoes, the entry fees—everything that makes these races cost prohibitive for many. He just ran his first IRONMAN 70.3

with another Racing for Recovery member, Chris. Behind the scenes, most outsiders would never guess that it's Andy's second time at Racing for Recovery; he lied extensively to me through his first. I'm not just a trained clinician—I abused substances for thirteen years. I know what I'm doing, I know when the program is working, and I know when someone isn't committed, no matter what words are coming out of their mouths. I can't choose sobriety for anyone—I'm here to listen and help when they're ready to make different choices.

For someone to go out of her way to stand up and lie about her sobriety in front of 137 people who need this—in front of parents whose kids have died, in front of people who are making the hardest and best choice of their lives—that's where I draw my line.

Everyone has that line.

It is very difficult when the people you love don't believe you or trust you when you've chosen sobriety. But how many times did you swear you weren't using? How many times did you say you'd quit? Knowing that you never have to drink or use drugs again, it's difficult when even kind people rush to reassure you that "relapse is part of recovery."

The hope, effort, love, time, and worry that our family and friends put into our sobriety is substantial, and it can cause them crippling grief if we do not choose to sustain it. You must choose sobriety for yourself, not your family, but understand that the consequences if you choose to use again include further collateral damage to your relationships and pain for the people who love you and are invested in your health and wellbeing.

Be secure in your conviction, and take this opportunity to build your self-esteem. Choose love—break the secrecy habits that you formed. Talk openly and honestly with your close friends and family. Harboring secrets makes you feel alone and vulnerable. Model choosing sobriety for yourself and for everyone watching you—you could save more lives than just your own.

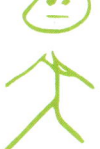

## WHEN WILL PEOPLE FORGIVE ME?

My greatest shame is the day that I chose to bring all of my rage into my home and family. I'll never forget the date—October 6, 1986. Instead of being in class at the University of Toledo, I'd chosen to be out drinking and drugging, completely disregarding the opportunity my parents had given me. When I staggered into my parent's home, my dad displayed courage and strength, as a parent who loved his son, by not enabling me. He confronted me. My stepmom, who had done nothing but try and love me, support me, and fill the void that was caused by my birth mother, also displayed courage by condemning my behavior. I responded with fifteen years of resentment, rage, and hurt, and I physically assaulted both of my parents.

The consequences of that choice shook my entire world. I damaged my relationship with my parents so badly that I did not think I could ever fully repair it. That should have been a major turning point in my life, but it took several more years before I chose sobriety, healing, and love.

When you choose something as monumental as sobriety and start building a different sort of life for yourself, it can be exhilarating. You're a new person, with new coping skills, doing all new things! For many people, it can feel unfair that the consequences of your past poor choices aren't wiped from your record—like you're being punished for someone else's crimes.

Some recovery programs promote this type of "rebirth" thinking, but it doesn't fit into what I know about addiction and sobriety. Although it can be difficult to face responsibility for the negative consequences of your past choices, it's the only option if you want to heal and grow. You cannot choose love and build your balanced, holistic sober life on dishonesty, and hiding from any trauma you caused will only increase the amount of trauma you carry with you.

Choosing love is accepting that you have hurt people, and that it will probably take more than words to rebuild your relationships. It is about making many right choices, forming good habits, and growing into the person you want to be. You cannot demand forgiveness, and you might not ever be able to reconnect with some people you've hurt. Choosing love isn't transactional—you can't barter making the right choices for guaranteed forgiveness. You can only work to become the best version of yourself, a person capable of loving and being loved in a healthy way.

With a lot of work, time, change and forgiveness, I did manage to rebuild my relationship with my parents. It is now full of laughter, respect, understanding, support, love, and pride! They're amazing grandparents to my kids and great in-laws to my wife Melissa. (Being a parent myself now to four emotionally healthy and stable kids, I can't imagine how hard parenting me must have been.)

Choosing love means having hard conversations that you'd rather avoid. It means starting those conversations and setting the tone. Talk openly with the people you love, and explain what you are healing from. Let them understand your pain, open the dialog, and reduce judgment on both sides. It's important to teach our families and friends why we did the things we did as we learn more about ourselves and our trauma. We need to make them understand that we love and respect them, and that we are committed to showing them that. They need to understand that the pain we felt was not their fault; that we hated ourselves, not them; that we do not blame them for it, and they should not blame themselves.

I knew when I got sober that there were many others who had feelings and opinions and had been affected by what I did. It's impossible to clearly see how your decisions are really affecting other people when you are still using, even if you have an idea that you're messed up. We have to explore what our choices did to our families, not to punish or shame ourselves, but so that we can be grateful that we are no longer creating that type of pain in their lives.

Avoid being combative. You need understanding to heal, but your loved ones need you to understand it is hard for them as well. Show them the compassion you want from them.

It's not usually a good idea to have these conversations when emotions are running high. Avoid creating more damage and misunderstanding by letting things cool down and giving everyone a chance to collect themselves and their thoughts— yourself included.

WHY DO I FEEL SO ALONE?

We have to build a lot of skills and resources within ourselves to heal and recover, but we cannot move on to the next steps before we choose love. The depressions that trauma creates are disconnective, and you won't heal from them if you keep yourself isolated and alone. To fix them, you have to reengage with people and look to connect in healthy ways. If you're still feeling alone, there's a few things you can do to jumpstart connections.

**FORGIVE YOURSELF.** The idea that people struggling with addictions are bad people is easy to internalize, fueling the cycles of self-destruction and low self-worth. Before you forgive yourself, you'll always be hiding something, and people can often sense that. Open the door to reconnecting with other people by recognizing that you are not a bad person and that you are someone worth having a full and honest relationship with.

**FORGIVE PEOPLE.** One reason we feel pain is because we hold other people's actions against them. This becomes a burden and can weigh us down. After many years of self-improvement, I have forgiven everyone in my life, even my mother.

Our societal systems and mindsets regarding addiction are based on the idea that punishment can prevent and stop substance abuse. Addiction typically stems from pain, and punishment only increases the pain the person struggling with addiction is facing. It can be difficult to work past the additional layers of hurt that people you loved caused you by shaming and punishing you, but if you want to reconnect, you have to forgive them.

**ASK FOR THE HELP YOU NEED.** A guy came to me the other day and said, "Todd, is there any chance you could help me get the tire to my bike fixed so I can ride it?" When I told him no problem, he was so grateful and surprised. I was excited that I could do something to help him out, but I was even more excited that he'd realized he could ask for help and that we were here to support him. That shows an incredible trust in your community, and it makes us all feel like we're in this together.

**TREAT EVERYONE WITH BASIC HUMAN CONSIDERATION.** I've heard some terrible stories of heartbreak and pain, but one of the saddest comments I can remember was when a guy in group said, "I can't believe people call me by my name here."

Think about that.

People are hurting that badly, all around us, and they're so disconnected that being called by their name seems remarkable.

You're not alone, even in feeling alone. There are so many people out there who are struggling with feeling disconnected and unloved. Show everyone you meet basic human consideration, and watch who blooms. You don't have to wait for someone to connect with you—make a huge difference in someone's life and connect with them first.

**LET OTHER PEOPLE BELIEVE IN YOU.** I had the concept for Racing for Recovery in my head back in 2001. It took fifteen years doing it, improving my education, getting licensed, staying the course, and ignoring whatever naysayer negativity was out there.

I'd just taken a tour of the building that is now the Racing for Recovery campus when a client came to me for help. At some point, he asked me what my plan was. I told him, and he pledged to help me rent the space to fulfill my dream. In a euphoric daze, I drove to the Thursday night support group meeting I'd been holding for fifteen years in a church and announced we were getting our own space.

Could I have insisted on waiting for a space until I could earn it all myself?

Sure, but my dream wouldn't be halfway as far along.

Choosing love means expanding your dreams to let other people contribute. It's collaborating and making something bigger together than you ever could apart.

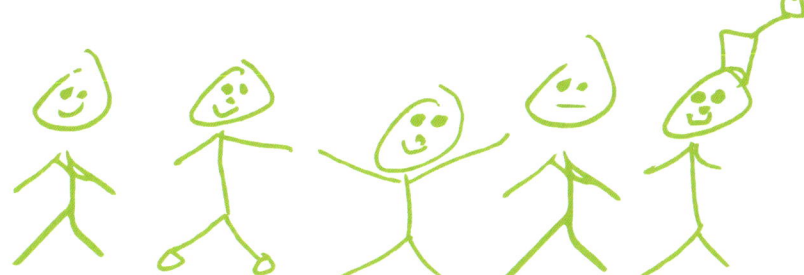

## HOW CAN I SAVE THE PEOPLE I LOVE?

When I was in the seventh grade, my friend Susan came by my grandma's house with her friend Annette. Annette was very, very drunk, falling all over and slurring her words. She threw up on herself, and we had to take her home in a wheelbarrow.

It scared me, but mostly, it made me sad for her. I wanted to help, but I wasn't sure how. Three of her friends were really worried about her. They took on the stress of Annette's behavior, even though they weren't making the bad choices.

A girl that I had an important relationship with for over seven years ended up having stomach ulcers from constantly worrying about me while I was using.

Addiction can impact people who never use. If you love or care for someone who is struggling with alcohol or drug addiction, you have to make tough choices too. If it feels like a situation you just can't win—well, that's because it is.

As soon as I heard the question, I was astonished I'd never been asked before: "Todd, do you get angry with people who don't get what Racing for Recovery is offering?"

I don't. Occasionally I get frustrated, because I want them to have what we have (it's awesome!). But I don't let it affect me personally; I use that frustration to motivate and guide my growth as a clinician. That way, the next time, I have new ways to convey our message and reach people who aren't able to hear it now.

Deep down, that frustration is really hurt. It bothers me that people suffer when I know they don't have to. But one of the things I learned early doing this, is that you have to control your own emotions. Everyone is responsible for their own emotions, so if I get upset over somebody else, that's a problem within me that I need to look at and address.

Recently, a client with two months of sobriety shared that her sister had picked her up from a Racing for Recovery meeting with beer in the car—then invited her to the bar. My client, who lost her father to drinking and messed up the lives of her kids and her family pretty badly for a while, went, and it was a struggle for her emotionally. She shared a lot of thoughts and feelings about how difficult it was watching her sister drink.

I was floored. "Hey, you've got to stay out of that bar. You're not gonna fix her. I've been doing this a little bit longer than you, and I wouldn't go sit in a bar and watch somebody drink right now. No way. It wouldn't be good for me, wouldn't be healthy."

I understood her motivations. She'd felt good for two months, and she wanted to fix her sister so she'd feel the same way.

I wish it worked that way, but it doesn't, at all.

You can't save anyone. I can't save anyone. We can be here to help, but we can't take on any of the suffering for them. There have to be some hard rules and boundaries in place. This is one of the hardest areas of addiction to navigate. The territory between enabling and support is fraught with obstacles, confusion, and hurdles. This is an area where making the right choice can feel so wrong until you are able to reason through some hard emotional truths.

**TRUTH #1: YOU HAVE TO SAVE YOURSELF FIRST.** Effective, healthy relationships come from both parties taking care of themselves first. If you are not healthy, you have nothing to offer. If you're coming into a situation that requires healing with your own emotional baggage, you will only hurt the vulnerable person that you love more. The kind thing to do is to work on healing yourself first.

**TRUTH #2: HEALING CAN'T BE OUTSOURCED.** As much as you'd like to take the pain away for the person you love, you can't. We're not capable. Each of us has to create our own sense of peace within ourselves. People struggling with addictions have to take responsibility for their own healing.

**TRUTH #3: THE CORRECT DISTANCE IS A BALANCE.** Often,

people are too supportive and drag themselves down. Other times, they are so distant that person in need feels abandoned. You help by staying out of the bar and having your loved ones come to you, not going to them, but you also have to let them know you're ready when they are.

**TRUTH #4: YOU CAN'T BE EVERYTHING TO ANYONE.** I have heard from many friends and partners of people in the Racing for Recovery community about how appreciative they are that they do not feel like they need to be—or even should be—the entire emotional support system for their loved ones. It is important not to make one person "everything" in someone's recovery.

It is frustrating to see friends and family continuously enable loved ones in their addictions, but again, I don't get mad at them. I just ask them to examine the results they're getting and suggest a different approach—one that helps their loved one to stop using drugs, rather than aiding them in continuing to use drugs. Counselors and therapists are trained to navigate these confusing issues and can help.

Friends and family can be very powerful when they express their love and support. Hearing words like, "Dude, I care about you and want you to live," can be the tipping point for someone to choose sobriety in transformation.

## WHAT DOES A STRONG COMMUNITY LOOK LIKE?

As we were walking out of a support group meeting today, one of the newer guys came up to me and registered admiration and some surprise—because I'd been in there to participate, not lead.

I had to laugh to myself about it later—of course I still participate! Man, I don't have all the answers!

I did not speak openly about addiction until I'd been sober for over eight years. I did not feel I had anything to say other than what a train wreck. When I decided to pursue helping others with my experience through addiction and recovery, I went back to school. I put the same tenacity into building a program that would truly empower people to create incredible sober lives as I had into destroying my own life with drugs.

At Racing for Recovery, I spend at least as much time listening as I do talking. It's not some conscious effort to be humble and stay grounded. Walking around here is humbling. I'm still learning, every day, from everyone I meet. That's a process that never ends. I will never know everything I want to know about recovery, because I want to know everything. This program has saved my life, over and over. It saved my life when it was just me and my running shoes; it gets that much better with each new person who joins and adds their perspectives and experiences

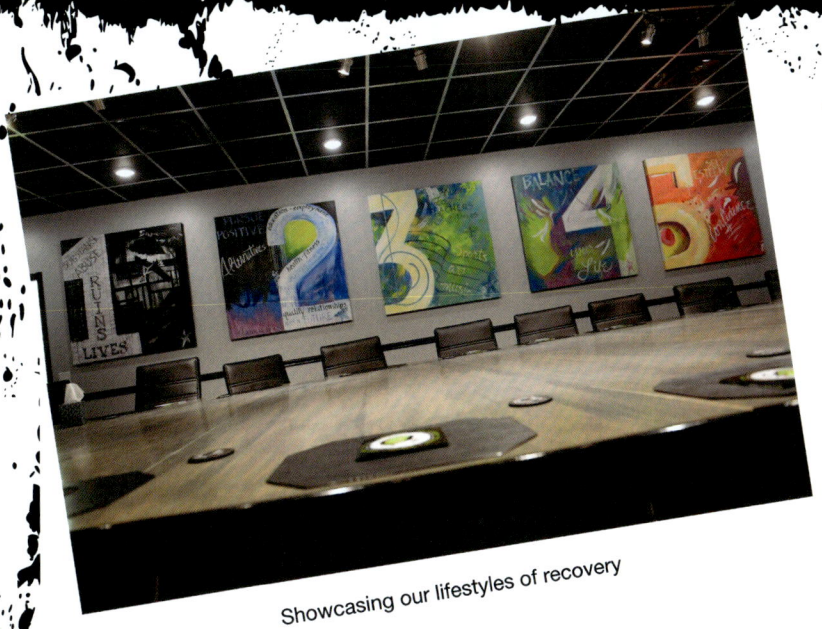

Showcasing our lifestyles of recovery

and talents.

We've built such a positive, unique, thoughtful community by believing in everyone from the moment they walk in the door. We welcome them and show them how incredible a balanced, healthy, holistic sober lifestyle can be. We invite them to utilize all of our resources and empower them to share their own talents. We make sure that people feel heard and valued, that we do not cultivate a victim mindset in ourselves or others, and that all of our stories are shared in productive ways. We work hard and search everywhere for techniques and theories that actually help people heal from trauma and live with inner peace. We've created a model that empowers everyone to play an important role, recognizing that helping others can be a powerful, inspiring way to improve your own recovery.

Some traditional recovery programs promote the idea of having one person who is further along in sobriety as your guide—a sponsor. At Racing for Recovery, we believe in having many people—a whole community of people—here to help you, because no one person has all the answers or support you need. We call these 'sober navigators.' When you connect with somebody, you bond with them, and they become part of your support system. We encourage people just to meet everyone in our community and start hanging out with them, building organic relationships. Conversely, when you're part of our community, if you see someone who needs help and you're capable of helping them, you help. By creating more balanced relationships, we've made a system of peers. No one is expected to have all the answers, and everyone is able to share their gifts—whether they walked in the door five minutes ago or they've been here since day one. As participants, we're all on the same level. We're a family with many questions and answers, looking for ways to say yes, make ourselves better, and support each other.

Sober navigators are there for support, but they also know they are not counselors—licensed, credentialed and educated clinicians—and do not try to be. When a problem becomes bigger than they can handle, they say so and refer it to a clinical level of care.

Every member of the Racing for Recovery staff has been helped through the program. The ten clinicians who have overcome addiction utilizing our program have more than eighty years of sobriety between us. Those who originally came in as clients built at least a year of consistent, productive, solid sobriety before we considered bringing them on staff. It's one of the ways that we show each other support and build each other up. I see someone who has turned their whole life into a series of awesome choices, someone committed to doing the right thing, even when it's the hard thing, who has that energy, that fire to help even more people on a deeper level. We'll do anything to support each other and give people the opportunities they need, from paying court fines to getting them licensed. We are a group of uniquely qualified counselors. Each of us can offer perspective, connection, and empathy as people who have been addicted to substances; we have all committed to and made incredible progress on the never-ending process of building healthy, balanced, holistic, sober lifestyles; and we are all licensed, credentialed, and experienced with the clinical side of recovery.

As the supervisory clinician, I do whatever I can to help make all of us better and more knowledgeable. Expanding my ability to help, from working with people in recovery to working with those who work with people in recovery, has been an exponential step for me. It's a great way to pay it forward and expand my impact beyond the people I'm in direct contact with each day.

As a team, we provide an ever-expanding amount of resources, from individual, group, and family therapy to support groups to fitness classes to housing. We help people find the access that they need to detox, medical appointments, dental appointments, case management. Some nights, between the people in the room and the participants online, over a thousand members of our community will be tuning in live to support each other and find the support they need.

We've never gotten a grant. We've funded everything ourselves, between billing for medical services, generous donations, and the proceeds of our annual 5k and book, merchandise, and movie sales.

We're flexible. We're forgiving. We're more concerned with how we can help and support each other than anything else. We'll make business decisions that don't make sense financially, because they're the right choices to make for healing.

I can't give you the ideal model community, because we still find new ways to make ours better every day. But it starts with choosing sobriety, choosing healing, choosing passion, and choosing love. It's a living organism made up of many other living organisms, but the principles are the same. The choices you learn to make in this book are the choices you need to make to build a strong community and a strong world. The results are beyond your wildest dreams.

## WHAT IF THE PEOPLE I'M CLOSEST TO DON'T BELIEVE IN MY PASSIONS?

By 2002, I hadn't touched drugs or alcohol in nine years. I'd finished playing semi-pro hockey, I was racing in IRONMAN competitions, I had a steady, sizable paycheck coming in, a lovely home, a beautiful wife and growing family, and I was so, so miserable. I was struggling so badly emotionally, I even had suicidal thoughts.

I was a broken soul. I was healing, but I was still very damaged. I was doing what everybody thought I should be doing: I got the job, the education, the house, the cars, the stuff! But it didn't mean anything to me. I still hadn't found myself.

When I found Racing for Recovery and realized it was my life's purpose, I knew I was going to do whatever I needed to do to make it work. I have an incredible sense of drive, and I devoted it all to Racing for Recovery. I had a purpose. I had a passion. I had a mission. And I was helping so many people.

What I didn't have was Melissa's buy-in. From her perspective, she'd married a suit-and-tie pharmaceutical sales rep who was making eighty grand a year, a guy who had a company car and life and health insurance; now, she had a husband who'd lost his job for starting a support group, four kids to feed, a house in bankruptcy, and repossessed cars. We didn't know how our bills were going to get paid and our lights were about to get turned off and, oh, by the way, I was jumping on a plane to China to do an IRONMAN.

For some strange reason, Melissa didn't believe me when I just told her everything was going to be okay. I knew I was rolling the dice, but I was positive how they were going to land. Even when nobody else could see it, it was so clear to me—and it really, really bothered me that my wife, of all people, didn't trust my vision.

I signed a book deal. I was so excited to tell Melissa I was going to have a book and it was going to help people; she just wanted to know what that would do for our family. When the television producers came to town to give Racing for Recovery its own show, they told Melisa she was going to be able to buy the house of her dreams. At the last second, the show got pulled. It was incredibly disappointing and painful, but the worst part was when my wife told me I'd failed her. I felt completely abandoned by her lack of support, and I could not handle that.

Abandonment was nothing new for me. I'd felt it since I was three years old—that was the hole in my soul created by my mom's suicide. Trauma doesn't build a tolerance the way drugs do. Trauma makes you more sensitive to the same type of pain. When you struggle with trauma like abandonment, compliments can feel much bigger than they are—like promises that you are good and safe and loved. On the flip side, criticism can also take on monstrous proportions. "I'm disappointed," might be the words that left someone's mouth, but they seem to mutate in mid-air; by the time your brain processes it, it sounds just like, "I'm walking out the door for good because you're the worst!"

Our marriage started to get bad in 2006, and it just got worse over the next few years. Melissa didn't trust me, but there were people who thought what I was doing was great. Naturally, I spent more and more time away from my family, working on Racing for Recovery and soaking up the support of people who believed in me and my vision.

By 2014, we'd filed for a divorce. I'd already been living out of the house for a year, in an apartment about half a mile away from my drug-days digs. All I could wonder was what happened to me—in sobriety, I'd had everything but my life's purpose; once I'd discovered my life's purpose, I'd lost everything else.

My wife had become my enemy. What I really couldn't understand at the time was that I had also become her enemy.

I was lucky enough to have the chance to figure it out. At the last minute, Melissa and I came together and decided we really wanted to recommit and save our marriage. We had to work on our communication, our understanding, and our perspectives. I realized I needed to choose to take my blinders off and look at things from her perspective. My wife wasn't doubting my drive—she was terrified to lose everything. I'd chosen to pursue my passion, and that was the right choice. But I hadn't recognized that I wasn't working on healing a portion of my trauma that twisted her concerns into attacks. I hadn't chosen to connect with Melissa and invite her to play a part in my life's mission. I hadn't balanced any of my choices with choosing love.

We completely turned it around, and saving my marriage is the most important thing I've done in sobriety. Learning to see things from other's perspectives and understanding and overcoming how profoundly my childhood abandonment affected my life was very healing for me. It was also a major catalyst for Racing for Recovery. Finding that balance put all of the pieces I'd learned about recovery together. It put me in the position to take everything to the next level. Just over a year later, we got the building. Everything changed and grew and became more than anyone could have ever imagined.

(Well, anyone else. To be completely honest, this is exactly what I knew it was going to be when I rolled those dice. I just couldn't see that it was going to be the result of choosing love and finding that balance.)

It took me about forty-five years of living, twenty years of sobriety, and watching my entire life start to crumble yet again to really dig deep and address how my childhood trauma was keeping me from choosing love. Once I started, though, I threw myself into it the way I've thrown myself into all my choices in sobriety, healing, and pursuing my passion.

Just like the choices we make in the other three categories, choosing love isn't a one-time deal. Honestly, I could live in a box and be just fine. Choosing love, though, meant understanding things from my wife's perspective. Once I was able to see it through her eyes, I got her the house that she wanted (the one those producers had promised her long ago) as soon as I was able. The result of that choice, for me, has been so much bigger and better than just having a great home. One of the many awful things about addiction is the guilt and the shame of all of the promises that you've broken and the people you've let down with your bad choices. Choosing love this time around, I'd not only taken care of my family, I'd done it by pursuing my life's work. Just thinking about it makes me cry a little. Nobody will ever really know how much achieving that goal means to me.

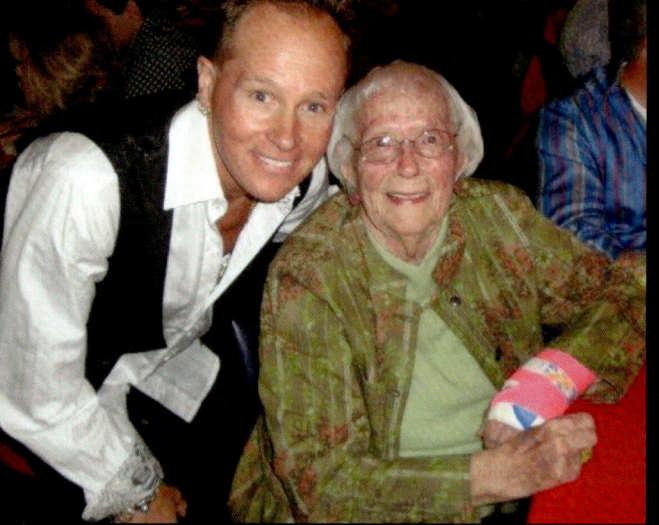

**MY CRAZY, KIND, FUNNY, INTELLIGENT FAMILY WHOM I LOVE DEARLY.**

With my Grandma. I would not have made it nor would there have been a Racing for Recovery without her endless support.

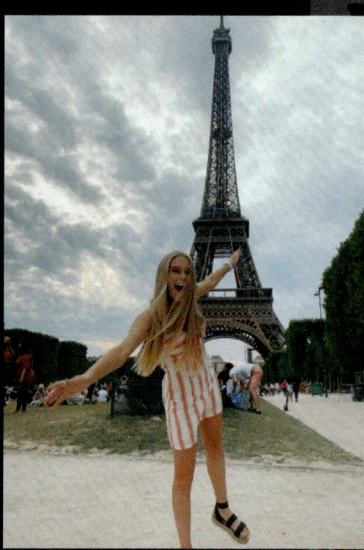

Madison in Paris, France 2019

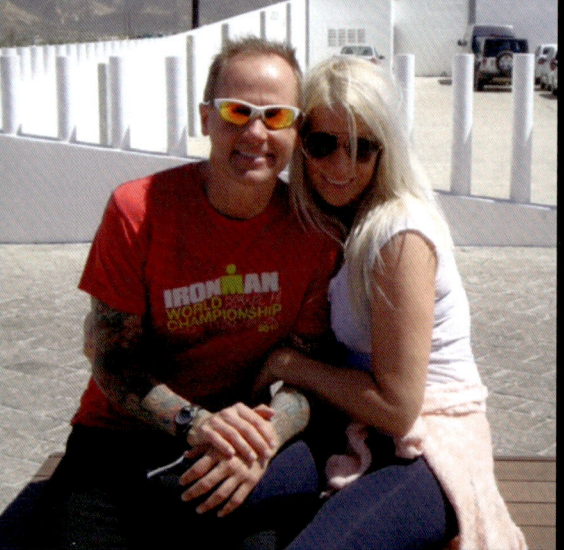

With Melissa at IRONMAN Los Cabos in Mexico

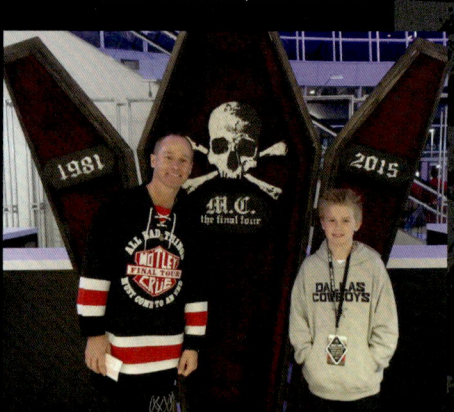

Me with Mason on the final Motley Crue tour in Los Angeles

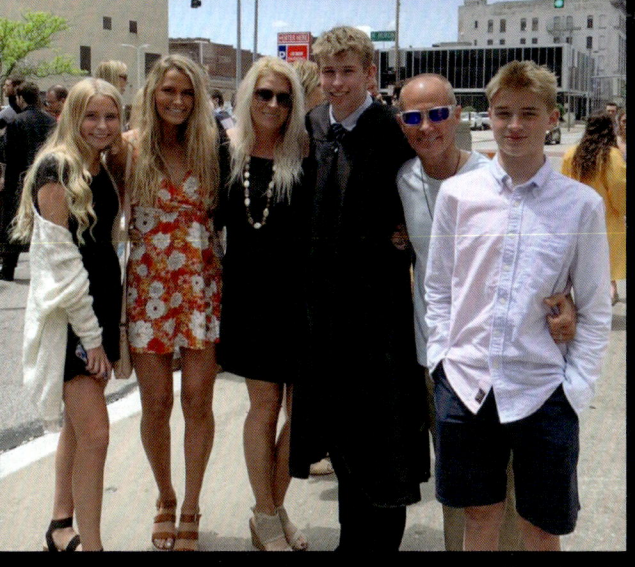

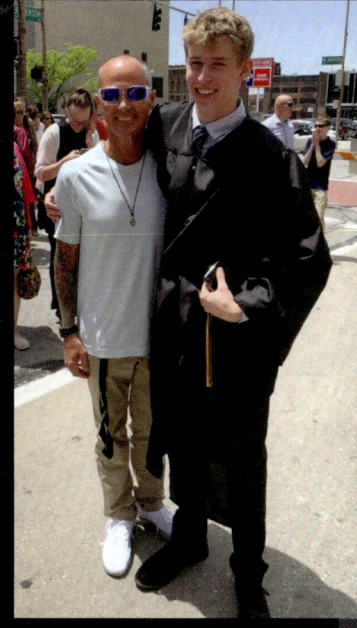

Konor's 2019 graduation

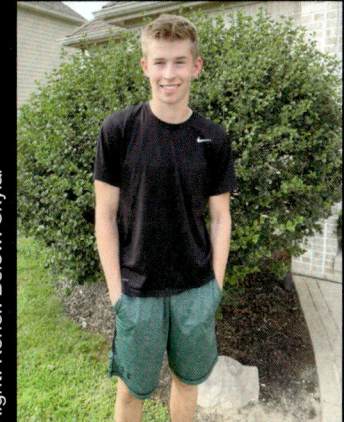

Right: Konor. Below: Skylar

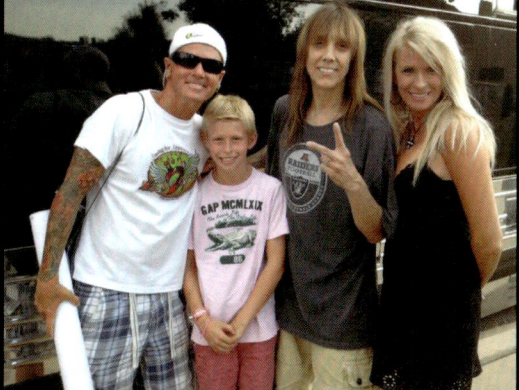

Me with Konor, Jeff Keith from TESLA and Melissa

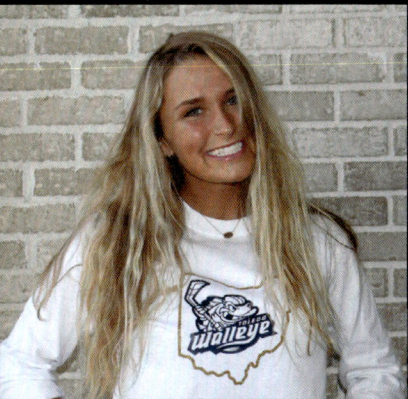

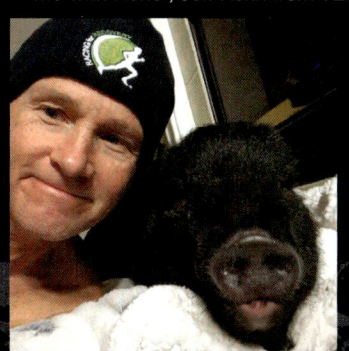

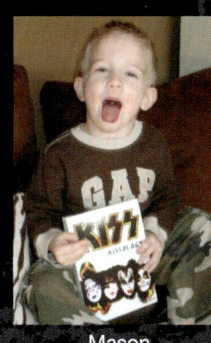

Mason

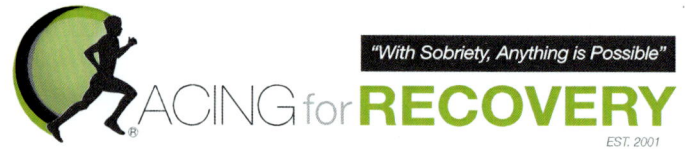

# INTERVIEWS

If each of us were building a house, choosing sobriety and choosing to heal would be like pouring the foundation of the awesome people we want to become. On that strong foundation, we build the amazing structures of the lives we want by choosing to pursue our passions and choosing love. Sobriety and healing are choices we make inside ourselves; love and passion are about building healthy connections with other amazing people and sharing our gifts with the world. The balance we strike between the four means everything. Never give up on your sobriety, your healing, your dream, or your love—that hard work will pay off, and you will prove to yourself and to the world that anything is possible.

I've given you a lot of examples of my bad choices and how I found my balance and made myself the luckiest guy in the world. Your path, of course, will look different from mine. Everyone's does! I swear, though, the formula will work as well for you as it does for me—choose sobriety, healing, passion, and love, keep them in good balance, and you're going to be the person you want to be. You're going to be happier, healthier, and live a better life than you can even imagine. The next five people you're going to meet will vouch for it.

I'm giving the last word to five incredible members of Racing for Recovery who have built lives that seemed impossible when they walked in our doors. They have all made very different choices from me and from each other, but they've made the right choices for them across the same four categories. Check out what the right decisions looked like for them, and let them inspire you—I know they inspire me!

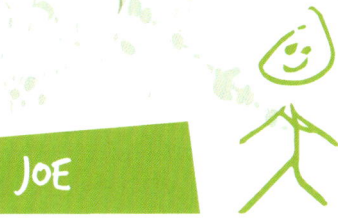

## JOE

When I was a kid, I felt like an outcast no matter where I was—in grade school, high school, and even a little bit in college. I felt like I never really fit in with anyone. I was always putting on a mask for everyone else. I was bullied for being fat, for being stupid, for the typical stuff that you encounter in school, and I always took it to heart. Now, none of that really bugs me, but I know back then it stuck with me because I always tried to be nice to people, even if I couldn't really relate to them.

Tim was one of my best friends. We grew up down the street from each other and went to grade school and high school together. We talked about everything. We also fought, the way friends do. One morning, we left football practice after we got in some dumb fight. I was trying to make up for it, and I distinctly remember saying, "Hey buddy, I'll see you tomorrow, love you," and he said, "Yeah, love you too man, whatever." That night, Tim passed away in his sleep. To this day, they don't know the exact cause.

I never really processed that grief. I cried, I commiserated with my teammates, but I never really dealt with the fact that, at some point, because I was really pissed off, I had wished he would die or go away. Then he did, and that was a big catalyst for a lot of the stuff that I got into from there.

I never opened up to other people or really connected with anyone afterwards. I didn't really have any solid relationships outside of my family. I had friends, but I didn't have close relationships. Going into college, I was still kind of in that funk, but I gained a reputation as a party guy. Whenever anyone went out with me, the next day, they were always going on about some crazy or dumb thing I did, and I realized that the crazier things I did while drunk or high, the more people seemed to want to spend time with me. I thought I was funny, so my life from college graduation onwards was an ever-escalating series of ridiculous events.

I was twenty-four or twenty-five when my parents told me, "You've got to go talk to someone, you're on a real bad path." My mom is a nurse, and one of her patients knew Todd. I went to one of his sessions every week or so, but from the time I was twenty-five until I was twenty-seven, I did the bare minimum. I'd show up and get my meetings in, but as soon as Friday hit, I knew I could get drunk or do whatever. I'd still have three days to detox and they would never catch it. I played the system, said all the right things, and didn't put in any effort. Sure enough, it was just a revolving door of me going back out and back out. I went through detox a couple times, and that didn't take. I was in a car accident where a primary factor was alcohol; the only reason I skated without any consequences was that I happened to know the cop that showed up.

My mom dropped me off at my apartment one time after I got out of detox. We had spent the whole night in the hospital, and when she left, she told me, "I'm done with you, don't call me unless you want help." In my head, I didn't know whether she was actually serious. She'd said something like that a couple of times, and it was always a pretty big hit. My parents have always been so incredible and supportive, and I thought I could probably schmooze my way back in. I thought, okay, maybe I need to get some help, but I was still kind of playing with the idea. Then my brother Alex, who is one of my best friends and someone I always look up to, said the same thing. He said, "I can't deal with you anymore, I'm not going to take your phone calls, I'm not going to take your texts until you go get help."

I took a shower, slept for about an hour, went back out, got more stuff, and came back and passed out. I woke up around three in the morning, still drunk, and looked around my apartment and thought, "Are you really happy? Is this what happiness looks like to you?"

It's true that you can't get sober for anyone or anything else; I had tried that numerous times. I tried to get sober for a girlfriend, for a job, but this time was different. Hearing my family really made me look at myself and ask whether this was the type of person that I wanted to be and whether this was how I wanted to live my life. I figured I had two options: keep going on the road I was on, which was just pain and darkness and probably a very ugly, early death, or I could choose sobriety. I didn't know where that was going to take me, I didn't know what was going to happen, but I knew that it had to be better. They gave me the push, but I just hated the person that I was and was becoming. It was really me saying, *"I can't live like this anymore."*

That was a big deciding factor in me finally checking in and going to Todd's IOP. I'd cycled in and out of Racing for Recovery for about three years before it finally stuck and I was continuously and consistently sober. I was ready now, and I went straight over to Todd's place, and they told me, "Go get detox, come on back, and we'll take care of you," and they have.

The trick was going in with an open mind. That was one thing I never did anywhere else. All Racing for Recovery asked was that when I came through the doors, don't use, and keep an open mind. I thought that sounded pretty easy and that I could do that.

The people there don't look down on you for what you've done, so I was really able to open up. Everyone really wanted to know what I wanted to do and how they could help me. No one in my peer group before Racing for Recovery had ever said, "That's awesome, what can I do to help you get there?" Having someone like Todd and my peers just believe in me; made everything click.

I think it's important to throw yourself into all aspects of it—the physical, the social, the spiritual, the mental, the emotional. As soon as I did that, as soon as I stopped worrying about how it looked or what people thought and said, "This is me, this is what I feel, this is what I need," the amount of support I was given was just a million times more than anything I could imagine.

The positive mindset and the happiness there are just contagious. Even coming in three days out of my last bender, I couldn't help but smile and laugh in that place. There's an energy in the room; you can feel it when you walk in. It's not just because of what they do, it's because of the people there. What helped me is finding other people who were putting in that work. I went out of my way to find people who were putting in the effort to be better each day. They helped motivate me to be better and helped turn my mindset from negative to a positive.

It's crazy now how much everything's improved. I guess I was always a really negative person before. No matter what it was, whether that was work or if we were going somewhere, I would just be negative. Now, it's easy to see the positive side of things.

I remember running into a couple at Racing for Recovery; they're married now, but back then they were just dating. She said something really nice about him, and I followed up with some snide comment. She said, "That was kind of mean, Joe, why would you say that?" That was how I had always talked to my friends and their girlfriends. I realized these people don't do that—they actually say nice things to each other and about each other.

There are a ton of people here who are always happy and smiling. They've been here forever and they stay here. At first, I thought that was kind of weird; now I see that they don't stay because they have nowhere else to go, they stay because they like it. If you go to another program's meeting, you'll see people who have been in the same chairs for twenty years, and they're still miserable. The people at Racing for Recovery aren't. They're always happy and positive; if they aren't happy and positive, they stick around long enough that they become happy and positive.

> I THINK THAT'S MY FAVORITE THING: YOU SIT IN THE SAME MEETING EVERY WEEK AND YOU SEE THE SAME PEOPLE COME THROUGH. WE TELL THEM IT GETS BETTER, AND AT FIRST, THEY'RE LIKE, "NO, I HATE THIS." THEN, ONE DAY, THEY INTRODUCE THEMSELVES, "HI, I'M SO-AND-SO, I'M JUST SO HAPPY TO BE HERE."

Being able to get stuff off my chest, it was like the weight got lifted and now I can feel empathy towards people and express those feelings. In a lot of my relationships, both personal and romantic, it was hard for me to express my feelings. I remember one ex-girlfriend describing me as having a wall up, where I would do all the stuff and say everything, but she said she never really felt like she knew who I was. Now, I'm able to be more honest about my feelings and express frustrations, and it's easier to connect with people. I have a great group of friends, and I'm currently in probably the best relationship of my life because I'm honest. I don't try to pull any punches about anything. I've learned a lot, and I'm more empathetic to people's feelings. When people have situations that upset them, it's easier for me to ask how I can help, and then act on it. I know now that actions speak louder than words.

My spirituality is being kind to other people and being able to connect with them. I get that spiritual component in my life by just being a good person now, being accountable, being relatable, listening to people when they need it. I guess my higher power or my thing that is greater than myself is my friends and my people. Just being able to talk to them, relate to them, and bring new people in, that makes my soul feel good.

It's insane to me how within about two years, my friend group now is comprised of people that old me probably wouldn't have associated with. I had this external projection of how cool or attractive my friends needed to be, because that's what I aspired to. Now, all that stuff really doesn't matter. I go meet new people, and I can tell pretty much right away whether people are genuine or fake. I try not to associate with fake people anymore. I really like people who are genuine and honest much better, even if they have their flaws. It's interesting to see how people that I associate with now embrace those and learn from those flaws.

No one's really had to be excised from my old friend group. My best friend, Jason, understands everything. He is on board 110%, and he's been good help. A lot of people recently started coming back into my life after they heard what I'd done or saw something on Facebook. They've been able to say, "Hey man, I'm really proud of you, that's awesome." I have yet to have anyone really question my sobriety. That was always one of my biggest fears getting sober, was that I would have to cut out all those groups of people. Initially, I had to step back, I needed to work on myself, but now we can go hang out and watch a band and no one questions it.

There are still a couple situations where they'll invite me to something and I'll choose not to attend, because it's just not the right thing for me. For example, my friends are going to a bachelor party, and they invited me. I didn't want them to feel like they couldn't do something because I was there, and I didn't want to feel like I was not a part of the group because I choose not to do what they do anymore. There's nothing bad about it, and everyone's really nice.

There are a couple friends that I no longer really talk to; it's not that I don't think they're good people, it's just that I don't do the things that they do. I've got a couple drinking buddies who I tried to go visit with after I'd been sober for a good six months. When I went to a summer party, it was fun, and no one questioned me, but it was one of those times I just realized this isn't for me. They're adults and they can make their own decisions, but they don't match up with my choices.

I'm not really a planner, but when it comes to sobriety, I had to have goals to reach toward. My first year, that was getting everything stabilized, making sure that my mental health was all in order, being more social, and developing friendships. My second year was focused on physical health, striving towards physical goals. I'll have two years of sobriety on June 6. After that, the next thing I'm going to focus on is mental challenges. I try to keep a balance between all of them—mental, physical, spiritual, and emotional—but I always like to put goals ahead of myself so I can keep working toward them. First it was just running a 5k, then it was a 10k, then it was a half marathon. Once we knock that out, we'll look for the next challenge.

During my addiction, I would get winded walking up stairs, and now I'm two weeks out from running thirteen miles in one go. My dad and I run every Saturday. If you would have told me I'd be doing that two years ago, I would've said you were out of your mind. I was only running if someone was chasing me. I was so out of shape. Now, when I lace up my shoes and go running, it's my way of decompressing and relaxing. If it's a nice day, I'll just go out and go for a run; I always feel better after it.

My diet has gotten a lot healthier. Before, I was basically just eating whatever I could get delivered to my house or whatever sounded good. That was one of the big changes. I lost about thirty pounds within the first three months of starting with Racing for Recovery. I'm much more physically fit, my diet is much healthier, and I'm in much better physical condition than I was back then.

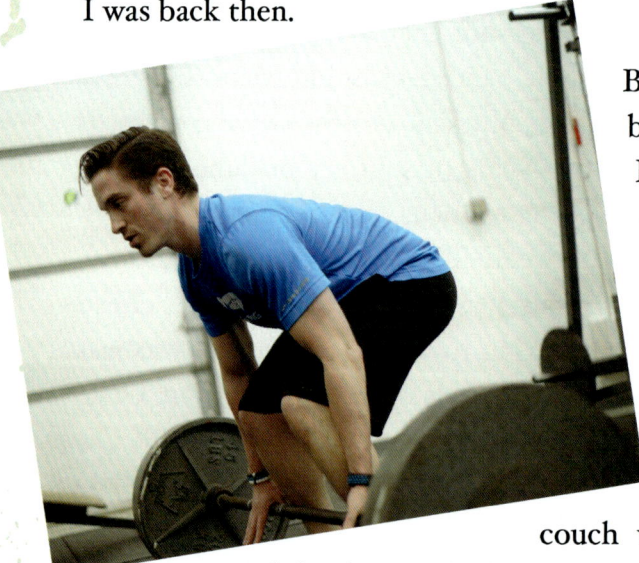

Building a routine, both in Racing for Recovery and outside of it, was essential for me. When I went home for the night, I knew I had to do something to progress forward, not just lay on the couch watching Netflix. It didn't have to be huge; things like eating breakfast every morning and trying to eat the same type of thing every week, are part of my routine that helps me stay on track. I know if I'm starting to feel kind of junky, or if I'm starting to have bad thoughts, I've just got to look back at my routine and reset everything.

I was always a big talker. I talked about a lot of stuff that I was going to do or that I wanted to do, and I didn't really ever put any action towards it. Being here at Racing for Recovery, these people taught me that actions speak louder than words. If I say I'm going do something, I have to do it. It taught me to be accountable. There's no more, "I'll get to that, I'll do that one day." Now, it's more like, "I'm doing this, I did this, I've done that, I'm working towards that by doing this now."

When I started seeing Todd, he'd ask me questions like, "Why don't you just go do things you want to do?" I honestly didn't know what I wanted to do. The things that I enjoyed—reading and writing, creating things, meeting new people and talking to them—a lot of people wouldn't think were prestigious careers, and that mattered to me. I was always pursuing someone else's dream of happiness, whether that meant going to college, getting a job, or something else.

My girlfriend bought me a journal for my birthday, and I've been using that to jot down ideas. When I was back in high school and even in college, I took a couple creative writing courses. I always enjoyed them, but it's never something I stuck with because everyone said, "That'll never go anywhere, don't do that, go do this." Now that I'm at Racing for Recovery, when I talk to people about it, they encourage me to do it. I've got a lot of ideas I've been jotting down, now I just need to get some time to sit down and actually type it. Once I get done with this half marathon, I really want to focus more on writing.

I think it's important for people to find things that they enjoy. You have to have other things to do, other things to focus on in sobriety. You have to have a balanced list of different things you can rely on. Writing down ideas I have for stories that I want to write is great. Just discovering new things is important. Todd told me to find something that I love doing and go keep doing it. For me, that's physical exercise, and now cooking—I used to hate cooking because it took too long for me to get food because I'd always start cooking when I was really hungry. Now that I can take time to actually cook and not have the danger of burning down the house, it's a great thing. I cook, I bake, I run, I write, I read all the time. I have to have a lot of different things to do because I don't ever want to be bored in sobriety, and am rediscovering things that I enjoy and finding new things that I enjoy. For example, I've developed a boardgame habit, where I'll just go find a new boardgame, and bring it over to people's houses. Just discover things that you love doing, and then do the hell out of them.

Racing for Recovery is a large part of my life, and it will always be a large part of my life. Todd is a wonderful human being. Everyone here is important to me, and they've embraced the people who are important to me. My parents are amazing, incredible people. I love them to death, and they are so involved in this movement. They come every Thursday and anytime they can show up, they do. For Thanksgiving this year, my family—my brother, his wife, my parents—all cooked dinner for everybody, over a hundred people throughout the day, morning to the night. It was great, I loved it.

> **TODD AND RACING FOR RECOVERY DIDN'T SAVE MY LIFE. THEY GAVE ME SOMETHING BIGGER. THEY GAVE ME THE ABILITY TO SAVE MY OWN.**

## TODD B.

I played sports my whole life; football, basketball, and baseball through high school, and baseball in college. I never drank, smoked, or did drugs through high school. I actually spoke at my old grade school for "Positive Addiction Week," because I was doing very well in high school and just never went down that path of alcohol or drugs. Sports were everything to me.

I went away my freshman year to school in Indiana. I was supposed to play football, but I blew out my knee my senior year in high school, so I ended up walking on in baseball. I made the team and started every game at third base my freshman year.

I didn't know a single person when I arrived, but I got invited to parties, and I started drinking and smoking every weekend and probably a couple of times during the week. I just chalked it up to a normal college, getting away, exploring, and figuring out life and doing things experience.

I ended up transferring because I wanted to try to play at a Division One school, and Indiana was Division Two. I walked-on and made the baseball team at my new school. During my third year in college, I had a collision at home plate with the catcher and dislocated my shoulder. I damaged nerves off of my spinal cord, lost feeling and function in my left arm for about three months, then came back from that and had surgery. That was kind of when I was first exposed to pain medication. I had been drinking and partying a little more, and used the pain medication to kind of amp up my night. I would pop a couple with alcohol, smoke some weed, and they just kind of became a little more regular. I ended up having three surgeries on that same shoulder over time.

I graduated with a bachelor's in education in 2001 and got a job teaching elementary phys ed for disabled students in public schools for four years. That was an unbelievable experience. I loved kids, I loved sports and fitness, and I really had a passion to help kids get physically fit. It was an awesome job. I truly cared about every single kid. I was up moving with them, playing the games, and it was really a lot of fun. I got engaged, got married, and got a house in Sylvania. Everything was going great, we were doing good and everything you're supposed to be doing in life. We got a dog. My wife got pregnant with our first child 2005; we've got three boys now.

We bought another house because we thought we had to get a bigger one, and got into some financial problems with that. I got laid off when they closed some schools down, which was very frustrating. I took a job as a mortgage loan officer for a year, which was a young, hard-partying environment. It was good money, but I didn't really enjoy it. It was just very stressful. I quit and got hired at a large manufacturing company in Toledo as a supervisor. I spent ten years there, continually moving up and increasing my pay. I was in the top 100 of the company, and they paid for me to get my master's degree.

At my core, I've just got this really incredible work ethic, so I was always working, even though there were other signs that I had a real problem all along the way. Freshman year in college, after that first night of really going out and partying, I was just kind of not aware of everything that I was doing. I had a really bad nosebleed, I was shaking, and I was really just completely out of sorts. I called my mom, kind of scared about what was going on, because I'd never felt like that before.

As a teacher, I was sober during the day, but after school I would drink, smoke, and pop pills. When I was working in manufacturing, I'd stop on the way home every single day, hit my one-hitter, smoke a little weed in the car. I'd stop at the gas station, get a few tallboys, drink those on the way home, then ask my wife what she wanted, pick up some more alcohol, drink that, smoke some more, popping some pain pills here and there.

I struggled a lot with my identity after I was finished playing sports. I'd identified as an athlete, and did pretty well at it. It's a very small percentage of high school athletes that go on to play college sports. An even smaller percentage go on to play at the next level, but I'd always dreamed of playing pro baseball. I was making good money at the time, managing a $23 million budget, but I couldn't handle my own home finances. I think that I was constantly trying to avoid that and myself.

If I had a bad episode with alcohol, I'd stop drinking and chill out for a little bit for the next couple days, just smoke weed. I lost my brother's Jeep at one point, so I said somebody stole it. I have no idea what happened, but we found it in another parking lot. I remember my family talking to me after that and kind of saying, maybe you need to tone this down and take a good look at yourself. I'd stop for a while, maybe wait until the weekend or a couple weeks, settle down from the last little episode. Then I'd decide I was good, and get back to life as normal.

It's scary to think about how many times I drove under the influence—pretty much every night. That was one of the bad choices that I still struggle with. We get so wrapped up in things that we think nothing's going to happen, and it builds this false sense of security. You make it home one night, so you think you can do it again, and "I'm not as bad as the last time." It's a horrible cycle to get into. It's hard to know that I was that arrogant, selfish, cocky, whatever word you want to use, to not only put myself in danger, but every other person on the road. It's absolutely disgusting to think about. It's embarrassing. I have a picture of a friend in my office. We used to bartend together, we started a personal training business. He died in a drunk driving accident. You would think maybe that would've reached me and hit home, and that I'd have made some changes, but I continued on. After he died, his picture was actually in my car, just kind of as a reminder, but I remember at one point taking it down and putting it in my glove box. I was embarrassed and guilty that I was doing what he did that ended his life.

On May 30, 2013, I went to some church guy's house to have a cookout. I drank prior to going over there, and drank another six-pack there. I left a little bit early and went to the bar about two miles from my house, drank some more by myself. On my way home, probably less than a half a mile away, I got in an accident, crashed into somebody. Thankfully, nobody was hurt. I got arrested that night and charged with OVI.

After the accident, I went to a place in town called Harbor Behavioral Health Care and had a diagnostic assessment. I lied through my teeth to them about how much I was really drinking and smoking and popping the pills. I got five individual counseling sessions with them, and at the end of the last one, the counselor gave me a piece of paper that had Todd Crandell's name and Racing for Recovery's name and phone number and some of the meeting times. I had never been to a meeting. In my mind, I had made up that meetings were a bunch of grumpy old dudes in a basement, complaining about their lives and smoking cigarettes. I thought, "That's not who I am," but my lawyer told me meetings would look good in the eyes of the judge, so I took a chance.

I went the next night and it was mind-blowing, totally different. I immediately felt like I wasn't alone. In our minds, we create the idea that how we use is normal, that everybody's doing it. I never did cocaine, never did heroin. I think I justified everything I was doing because it was socially acceptable. Anywhere you go, people are drinking, and I honestly think that alcohol is probably the biggest problem we have. I know you hear a lot about the opioid epidemic, but alcohol is at every single corner you pull up to, every restaurant, movie theater, sporting event, whatever. It's just always there, and it's normal. Marijuana is becoming the same way.

Early on, I remember thinking that I'd gotten in trouble because of alcohol, so I just needed to stop drinking. I kept my marijuana and my pills and pipes, and thought, "Maybe I can just smoke weed, that'll be cool." I had thought about moving up to Michigan, growing my own weed up there, since it was legal, and smoking on my front porch until the day I died. I didn't think I wanted to live without drugs or alcohol, didn't think I could. Racing for Recovery started to show me that you can.

There's two things that Todd said early on to me that impacted me a lot.

> **YOU NEVER HAVE TO DRINK OR USE DRUGS AGAIN; THAT'S A FACT. THE SECOND ONE WAS NOTHING GOOD CAN COME IF YOU DRINK OR USE DRUGS AGAIN, AND THAT'S ANOTHER FACT.**

I really kept those two things in my mind, knowing that, when I did drink or use, I struggled, and bad things would happen. I said, "Alright, I'm going to give this a chance for a while and see how things go."

Coming to Racing for Recovery meetings, I realized that it doesn't matter what you're getting drunk or high on, it's self-destructive behavior. It's all related. We're numbing ourselves from something, and that's a problem. We're meant to experience everything in life, feel everything—emotions, pain, all kinds of things. If we're putting something into us or if we're doing something to ourselves, whether it's cutting, shopping, gambling, or whatever, those are all bad things, and we shouldn't be doing any of those. I got rid of my pipes, marijuana, pills, all that stuff. I never drank or used another drug after that car accident. **My sobriety date is June 1, 2013.**

I lived in Sylvania, and so does Todd. Even before I knew him, I'd always see him around, biking and running. I remember back in the day, I would drive in to get some shitty food at McDonald's on a Saturday or Sunday morning after a long night partying, and

I'd see Todd running, and just think, "Look at this guy, shirt off, sunglasses on, thinking he's some badass." I was a few months into being sober, driving down that same road, and there he was, running. I couldn't believe how much had changed, and how grateful I was for what he was showing me.

> **I PULLED MY CAR OVER, GOT OUT, AND JUST WENT UP TO HIM AND GAVE HIM A BIG HUG.**

There are so many different things that I've done in sobriety that I never thought I would, like going to my first wedding sober, going to baseball games sober. I went to my first concert sober just this past summer, Pearl Jam in Boston with Todd and two of our other staff members. He had helped a family out there and they got us a suite at Fenway Park; it was unbelievable. There are different things I've always wanted to do that I didn't trust myself enough when I was using. When I turned forty and hit five years sober, I bought a motorcycle. I grew up on dirt bikes and four-wheelers, and I love to ride. I got my concealed carry gun license, too. I'm good, I'm confident, I'm comfortable. I take guitar lessons from a woman that comes through here—there's just all kinds of things that I'm exploring, doing, and enjoying now that weren't options before.

It's a totally different world now, with a clear mind and being able to deal with everything emotionally. When I was drinking and getting high, I was doing all the right things: getting a job, finishing school, getting married, having kids, getting the house, the stuff you're supposed to do. When I got clean and sober, I lost a job, lost the house, my wife had four miscarriages, we had deaths in the family, but I didn't drink or get high or do any of that stuff. The bad things, we deal with. We are not immune to life's hardships, and we don't have to drink or use because of that. We're supposed to feel everything; the good, the bad, the difficult, the pain, the hurt, happiness, all of those; and every one of those emotions is more intense with a clear mind and body. It's amazing to experience all of that.

With all the stuff that I have done to my body throughout my life—sports, working out a lot, lifting weights, a lot of manual labor for my brother's company, and I'm just a bullheaded dude that always tries to do everything myself—I started to have a lot of back problems. I'd always gone to the doctor to get some steroids and painkillers, but I kept choosing to do the same stuff. I continued for so long that it caused structural damage. Two years into my sobriety, I had to have major back surgery.

In one meeting, a gentleman named Scott said that he'd had surgeries without any pain medication. I was like, wow, every surgery I've ever had, I've always sucked down all the pills they gave me and then got more. It just kind of stuck in my head, this guy did them without it, and I told the doctors about my history and that I wanted to recover without the meds. They told me there was no way, that I'd need them.

I spent four days in the hospital, recovering on intravenous medication, but when I was released, they wrote me a prescription for 160 pills, and I didn't use a single one. They wrote me off at work for twelve weeks, and I was back to work in two.

> **I WAS FINALLY ALLOWING MYSELF TO FEEL THE PAIN AND THEN ADJUST WHAT I WAS DOING, RATHER THAN COVERING IT UP.**

Our bodies are very smart and intuitive and are speaking to us constantly, and we just need to be open to listen to what's going on. Feeling pain in my back, I stopped to evaluate what I'd been doing, and tried to adjust it going forward, so I don't have that same pain. It's similar to addressing any kind of problem we're dealing with, whether its financial or relationships. It's the opposite of how we try to deal with things with addictions.

I remember going to get my staples out, and I'm wincing and making some noise, and they couldn't understand why the meds weren't working. They were just shocked and amazed when I told them I hadn't taken anything the entire time beside Tylenol and Advil—all because one guy planted a seed in my head, and I started to believe that I could do that.

I shared that story with Scott and thanked him just a few weeks ago. He had no clue what impact him sharing in a meeting had on me. You never know how communicating your story impacts somebody else. Without Scott, maybe I would have used them. Maybe I would have gone right back down a bad path. But I didn't, and good things continue to happen.

I was on antidepressants, pain medication, allergy medication, a maintenance inhaler for asthma, and an emergency inhaler for asthma. With my sobriety, I ended up not having to use the antidepressants anymore or the painkillers.

I had exercise-induced asthma since high school. I was always using the emergency inhaler during sports and I started that maintenance inhaler probably in early college. I smoked cigarettes for a long time, which didn't help, but I quit on my oldest son's first birthday, while I was still drinking and doing the other drugs. I asked my doctors if there was anything else I could do to help, because it was like $300 a month for my maintenance inhaler. They said, "Oh, not really." They didn't even go down the path of changing my diet.

Dairy causes a lot of mucus and phlegm and inflammation, and the things that meat and animal products do to our bodies internally aren't good. Learning more and talking to Todd, I decided to give a plant-based diet a shot and see what happened. January 1 of this year was the last time I ate any animal products, any meat or dairy. Probably six weeks into it, I got pretty bad chest congestion; my breathing was really bad. After that, everything got so much better. In less than three months, I was able to stop using allergy medicine and the inhalers. It feels awesome, being able to breathe for yourself.

I came to Racing for Recovery in 2013, and I will forever come to meetings, and am forever grateful for what I've learned and have been taught here by Todd and the program and other people. I've been really involved since the day I walked in, and I joined the board of directors and tried to raise funds and help grow the organization. Todd talked about how he'd love for me to come on board and help him more with Racing for Recovery, but there really wasn't an opportunity. I had a wife and three kids, I couldn't just make a leap without a plan.

In January 2016, we toured this building, and realized it was amazing, everything we wanted. That April, I was laid off with six months severance, so I had a chance to really think about what I wanted to do with my life. I had several job offers, including a dream job at my old high school with tuition reduction, a good salary, an opportunity to do something that I really would have enjoyed, great healthcare benefits and things like that.

I turned it all down to follow my heart to Racing for Recovery—for no money, no health insurance, and not a clue really, what we were going to do. It was just basically three guys giving it our all and seeing what happened. It's unbelievable what has changed and what has come about in just three years. Every year, we're helping more people every day, adding more meetings, more fitness activities and groups and staff members. It's the passion, the care, and the drive that we have. You can't duplicate it, you can't teach it. It's something that Racing for Recovery and Todd has been able to offer all of us.

What one of his choices, twenty-six years ago, has done for so many people is unbelievable. He often says, "I just want to make this work. I just want to keep going. I want to make a difference." I'm going, "Dude, you're looking at one of them."

> IT'S CHANGED MY LIFE, MY FAMILY'S LIFE, IT'S JUST UNBELIEVABLY AWESOME TO BE A PART OF IT. I CAN'T IMAGINE DOING ANYTHING ELSE NOW FOR THE REST OF MY LIFE.

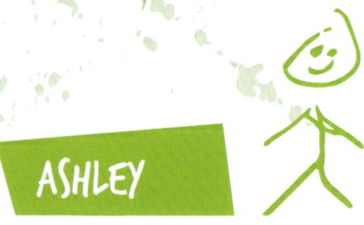

When I was young, my dad was a pastor, and we had a huge church split. I think it's hard for people that aren't religious and really deep into church to understand why that's a traumatic thing, but I had adults coming up to me and my sister when we were children, telling us why they didn't like our parents and how horrible they were. One of the church members cornered me in a restroom stall one time and just lay into me.

My mom has MS, and the illness itself put a lot of stress on our family when I was growing up. It put a lot of stress on her, and because I was the one closest to her, she just kind of made me her target. She was very emotionally and verbally abusive, and that took a toll. Nothing I ever did was good enough. If I brought home a good grade or did something notable in the band or choir, there would usually be some kind of a compliment, but it was always laced on the back end. When I hit high school, it just escalated. She would make comments about my weight all the time. She would tell me that other people had said things about my weight when really it was just stuff that she wanted to say to me. I watched her yo-yo diet, and the way that she talked about nutrition and then talked about weight made me really self-conscious. I was so withdrawn they thought I was using drugs. I wasn't; I was just so unhappy, so anxious, and so depressed, and they just weren't listening to me.

The crazy thing is that my mom has a background in psychology. I think that people who are psychologists and work in the mental health profession can be the worst with dealing with their own families.

I was displaying all of this hurt and these cries for help. I slept horribly all through high school. I couldn't sleep. I wouldn't be able to sleep until four or five in the morning, and my mother just wasn't getting it. She would say things like, "We need to keep you on your sleep schedule," and "You just need to go to bed earlier." My junior year of high school, I really started to put weight on. I was stress eating. My parents would go to bed, and I would go into the kitchen and just eat because it made me feel good. I was so hurt and so desperate to just get some relief, and that was helpful to me.

I went away to college, but I wasn't emotionally prepared to be there. I slept through classes and was just deeply depressed and not present. I came home after the first year and things were just terrible. My mother would scream at me and tell me she hated me. She would slam my door. I remember one time, I was sitting on my bed in the corner of the room, backed up in the corner in the fetal position, just asking her to back off and give me some space, and she wouldn't do it.

I was really involved in the church we ended up going to after my dad's church. The church I grew up in, the Church of Christ, they don't use instruments for worship. It's really conservative and women can't really be involved, so when we went to this new church, I jumped at being in their worship. I got really close to the worship pastor and his wife, and they actually let me move in with them to get away from my mom. The worship pastor's wife was so understanding and really listened to me. She was the first one to really believe me and listen to me about all the stuff that had been happening with my mom, so I kind of viewed her as a mother figure.

The pastor's wife actually ended up sexually abusing me for a year and a half while I was under their roof. I think she saw my vulnerability, and so she just preyed on me. I didn't talk about it to anyone. She never threatened me with violence or anything like that, but she knew me. I'd opened up to her, and she knew that just the fear of repercussions, or even that it would hurt her was enough to keep me quiet; I don't like anybody to hurt as a result of anything that I do. She would just threaten me with that and remind me, "If you ever tell anyone, they're going to know, and you're not going to be able to play at church anymore." and "It's going to affect me." She framed it like we were in a relationship; up until six months ago, when I actually started dealing with that specific piece of my past, that was still how I thought about it. I had blocked and shut down all of that sexual abuse and how it got started.

I got drunk for the first time when I was nineteen, living with the pastor and his wife. I was so stressed out. She had a lot of mental illness she wasn't dealing with, and I was trying to manage her and help her. I watched her hide booze in her house and drink. I wanted to fit in with her, but then, when I really drank for the first time, I discovered wow, this actually helps me manage this. That's kind of how I thought at that time: not that it was shutting the emotions down, but that it made me feel better. My eating ramped up, and the drinking became a new factor.

I finally got out of that situation a year and a half later. She actually ended up moving out of her house and coming out, so she stopped it. She still would kind of come back to me here and there; we still kept in contact. Up until about two months ago, she was still an active part of my life. I've been married for about seven years, and in the first couple weeks my wife and I were dating, I made a point to tell her about this woman because she was still actively involved with my life on a friendship level.

I'd started drinking, but my drinking didn't really get intense until I started professionally gigging as a musician in 2013. I had so much anxiety, and drinking helped me manage huge crowds and rowdy people. I would get there and have a double cocktail and a shot before I even started, and that established the trend for the entire night. The drinking just picked up from there; it went from just on the weekends at gigs to during the week when we would go out, and then I got to the point where I was drinking at home by myself. I met my wife (the most amazing human being in the entire world) in 2010 and got married in 2011. We were in our early twenties when we got together, so she saw this whole metamorphosis in me.

Actually, when we met, I hadn't come out yet publicly. Three weeks after we started dating, I was pulled out of the closet by the church by another pastor's wife. She'd been purposely looking for information on me, and she found my Yahoo! Personals page. I got a call from one of the church leaders, and he said, "We saw that you have this dating profile, and it says that you are into women." At this point, I was living two lives, which is really stressful, and I was so sick of not being authentic that I "fessed up."

This church ended up telling me that I was no longer allowed to be on the stage, and that it was probably better that I found another place to worship; when I decided to "change my life," they would "be there" for me.

My parents didn't know I was a lesbian yet; they had actually moved to Alabama by this time, but I knew if I didn't tell them quickly, they would find out from one of their friends from this church. I couldn't even wrap my mind around the idea of telling my mom. In the church I grew up in, being gay is just a sin, and it's not okay. As a psychologist, my mother understands that your sexuality is not something that you choose, but because she so firmly believed what she believed about the Bible, she thought gay people just needed to be single for life.

My wife helped me come out completely. She sat in the living room with me while I typed out an email to my mom. When I sent that email, things were bad for a while. My mom was just really horrible and would point out how I was walking the wrong path. I did bring my wife home with me for Christmas, and they weren't rude to her, so I was relieved. Even though I know my mom still feels the way that she does, they respect my wife and our relationship, and they always have, so that's good.

I'm very confident in my sexuality now and I don't feel like I need to hide it from anybody, but there are still things in the back of my head that I was always told: "You're going to hell," and "Who you are is not okay." That voice was loud, even through adulthood, and it wasn't limited to my sexuality. I know that none of the sexual abuse was my fault, but I still have in the back of my head, "You had so many opportunities to put the brakes on this." I dealt with some ADHD: "Who you are is not okay. You get too wrapped up in things. You're not focused enough." It was never, "You aren't focusing right now," it was, "You aren't focused enough, you are irresponsible, you're lazy, you aren't feminine enough." That was basically the voice's recurring refrain: "Who you are is not okay." I developed this intense fear of people not approving of me and desperation for people's approval, and that led into issues throughout my life of not advocating for myself and not speaking up when I'm not okay with something.

I was so anxious and depressed, and I was on a whole cocktail of anxiety medications. I was on the highest dosage of one that you take daily for maintenance, and then I was also prescribed Xanax and Klonopin at different times. The psychiatrist was actually convinced at one point that I had a mood disorder, so she threw in a mood stabilizer, and I was just miserable. I was drinking heavily on top of the medications, and I got to the point where I was blacking out at the end of gigs and still driving. I drove drunk all the time from our gigs. I didn't think that there was an issue with my drinking because in the music community, drinking heavily is normal. I was just living in my unhappiness. Everything that I had going on just continued to amplify.

The crazy thing is I'm always perceived as a really positive person, really upbeat and optimistic, and while that's true, I think I manufactured or amplified that part of me because I was so used to feeling like an inconvenience. Growing up, if I showed emotion, it wasn't a good thing. My mom would tell me, "You shouldn't feel this." If I did let things slip and I was real with someone, they wouldn't want to be a part of my life anymore. A couple years ago, I could have been having the worst day or feeling suicidal, but if you asked me how I was doing, I would have told you I was really great. I liked being that person that made people smile, so my friends in the music community thought I was really, really happy. Now I can tell them I was miserable. I got up to 446 pounds at my heaviest, and I'm a 5'3 woman. I could hardly stand for more than thirty seconds without my legs starting to shake and my lower back seizing up because I was holding so much extra weight.

I was in cognitive behavioral therapy and I just happened to mention alcohol to the therapist. She asked me how much I was drinking and I told her. She said,

> **"YOU DO REALIZE THAT THAT'S NOT NORMAL,"**
> **AND I REALLY DID NOT—THE THOUGHT HAD**
> **NEVER OCCURRED TO ME.**

In my mind, l wasn't drinking nearly as much as my other friends in the music community. I wasn't counting the alcohol that I was drinking at home by myself to manage my emotions. She had me track when I was drinking, how much I was drinking, what the day was like, and what the circumstances surrounding the day were like. It was crazy, until I saw it on paper, I didn't realize how much of an issue it was.

One of the days that I tracked, we went to a friend's album release party. I had five or six drinks before we got there, and I hadn't even eaten. Then I drank the entire day. The thing that finally scared me was the following week, when we were driving home from seeing a friend's play and I went up on the curb. I got to therapy that Friday and we talked about it a little bit more extensively. She was familiar with Racing for Recovery, so she recommended that I check it out.

That Saturday, I drank heavily. I woke up Sunday morning, and I quit. I don't know what switch flipped inside of me; I think having it pointed out to me, finally realizing there was an issue, and just being so tired. **October 15, 2017 was the first day I got sober, and I went into Racing for Recovery for my assessment.**

I think what Todd does with IRONMAN and stuff is really cool, but I didn't have that whole starstruck thing. I was drawn to this program because I'd read his background and all he went through. To know that he went from being so broken to where he is now, that appealed to me. I wanted what he had.

When I walked into Racing for Recovery, I was so terrified, because I knew that they were going to want me to open up. I sat in my car before I walked in and had a mini panic attack. The first session, I went in and met with Todd, and he told me that he was proud of me for walking in there, and that blew my mind. My mom hardly ever told me she was proud of me, and definitely not proud of me for just existing as a human being.

Every person I talked to was incredibly warm and caring and very non-judgmental. I was kind of skeptical at first, because I've seen people play like they're non-judgmental, when in reality, they really aren't, but nothing I said shocked them at all. I have not seen intolerance at all. I've never felt like anybody has treated me any differently or treated me less than because of who I am or what my sexuality is or any of that. I think that's part of the beauty of all of us being there—

> **BECAUSE WE ALL HAVE HARD STUFF IN OUR LIVES, THERE'S A LOT LESS OF AN INCLINATION TO JUDGE. I'VE NEVER FELT ANYTHING BUT LOVED AND SUPPORTED AND ACCEPTED THERE.**

I'd developed such intense trust issues, and I still struggle sometimes verbalizing things, but I was able to open up, and be vulnerable about what was going on with me a lot faster than I think I would have been able to with a lot of people.

I never got a DUI or anything, I never had any like legal consequences, and my drinking didn't affect my marriage. I wasn't court-ordered, I'd 100% chosen to be there, so I thought, "You can't do what you do most times, where you share information, but also try and make it seem like it's not that bad. You just need to lay it all out there." I was very honest with Todd and very honest with my assessment. I had been taking a medication for sleep called trazadone, a pretty intense sedative, and I told AJ that I would drink, and then come home and take that to sleep. He said, "You do realize you're very lucky to be alive, because a lot of people don't wake up the next morning after they combine those two?" He pointed that out to me, but it didn't feel judgmental—it was helpful and more confirmation that I really needed to be here, that this is something I really need to be doing.

Todd just listened to me and what I wanted. When I started to examine it, I realized I just really wanted to understand certain aspects of myself, and why I respond to things certain ways. I started on this journey to be a better human being and like myself more. It wasn't like everything hit at once, things were just very gradual. Everything that he's recommended to me, even if I haven't understood it, I've tried it, and I've seen the benefits from it. That's enhanced my trust in him as someone that I can always be completely honest with. I can ask his advice about things, because I know he'll never tell me what to do, but he's always going to recommend something that's going to be helpful. If he won't answer my question, it's because he wants me to answer it.

> **I THINK A MISCONCEPTION IS THAT BEING INVOLVED WITH RACING FOR RECOVERY MEANS YOU HAVE TO BE TRAINING FOR A TRIATHLON OR EVEN BE HEAVILY EXERCISE-FOCUSED.**

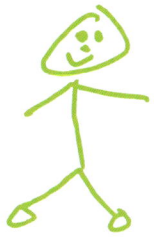

When I came in, I wasn't even really exercising consistently; they meet you right where you are. They encourage exercise as part of the healthy, holistic, balanced lifestyle but they make it very clear that you absolutely do not have to be doing that to be involved or to feel involved.

We talked about my physical goals. Todd encouraged working out in general because, physical benefits aside, it's very good for mental health. I started working out pretty regularly and establishing that routine.

I've lost about 200 pounds from my highest weight. Physically, I feel a lot better. I started running three or four months ago, which I never liked to do. I run first thing in the morning, and it's kind of like natural Xanax for me. For the rest of the day, it just kind of chills me out. Sports was one of the things that my mom used as a weapon. I was really involved with soccer in elementary and junior high school and even early high school. I was playing indoor soccer with this co-ed league, but when I started to put on a little weight, my mom told me if I didn't lose it, they were going to pull me out—completely counterintuitive, because it was the thing I was doing for exercise. But she did pull me out of indoor soccer, so I lost that thing that I loved. That's kind of when the exercise tapered off for me. To now have that back in my life, not in an organized sports sense, but to be in control of that aspect of my life, that's pretty cool.

I run four days a week. The other two days, I'm either on the elliptical or the bike, and I take a solid day to rest every week. When I started running, I was going out seven days a week, and Todd told me that was not a good idea. He advised me how to build it up. When I started on the treadmill, I was doing nine minutes of walking and one minute of running, and then repeating that three times. I stepped it up thirty seconds each week until I finally hit a mile. Now, I pretty much run for forty-five minutes solid. My goal is to do a 5k. The first one I'm going to do is through Racing for Recovery in October, so my main goal was just to build it up to 3.1 miles. I can run two and a half miles now, so I'm getting there.

I discovered that on the days that I work out, my mental health is like a hundred times better. Todd recommended I go out and exercise first thing in the morning, before I do anything else. I was a little skeptical, because I don't like to wake up very early at all. Musicians are not morning people. But I discovered that it changed the course of my day. I found out that, while I do need to have one rest day a week, it is very important, even on my rest day, to get up and do something. It just has this natural calming effect, which snowballs when I encounter stress throughout the day. My nervous system is so much more calm, so I'm actually able to think a lot more clearly. Before I was exercising, I had so much pent-up anxiety that had nowhere to go.

I had been curious about the plant-based diet because I've always struggled with what happens for animals to get to your plate. When I found out that Todd was vegan, I just asked him if I could spend a session asking him a bunch of questions about being vegan. At no point did he put pressure on me; he just answered all of my questions, gave me some recommendations about some documentaries to watch and things to read, and told me that if I had any more questions, to let him know.

I watched one documentary on Netflix called *What the Health*, and I just knew what I needed to do, and I treated it just like my drinking. We still had cheese in the house, but I quit eating meat that day, and then a week later, I was completely plant-based. I just went completely in with it and definitely saw the health benefits. If you just looked at my blood work, you would think I'm a lot smaller than I am. I think coupling the vegan diet with not drinking and not utilizing marijuana is what helped me to get off of my medication. I'm a total nutrition nerd now. I soak up reading about that stuff and listen to podcasts all the time.

Racing for Recovery promotes healthy eating and treating your body well, however you choose to do that. There are people taking all sorts of different nutritional approaches there. For me personally, plant-based was the way to go. It fit in with my set of ethics, and I knew it was the best thing I could possibly do for my health and my body. Going vegan fit perfectly into the sobriety process for me, because I spent so much time being absolutely terrible to my body, and I saw this as a way to be good to my body. I started to like myself a little bit more and be a little easier on myself.

I went out and saw a plant-based nutritionist on my own, just because I wanted to fine-tune things more, and that was important for me. The nutritionist doesn't just focus on the eating changes, she focuses on the emotional aspect of it, which really fit in beautifully with my journey at Racing for Recovery. She worked on helping me develop a healthy relationship with food, and she's still available to me when I need to ask her questions or if I'm struggling with something. She never gave me a specific meal plan, but taught me the things that are good for me to consume and why.

When I started going to Racing for Recovery, I was still on all of that anxiety medication. About three or four months into sobriety, when I'd been vegan for two months, I went in to see the psychiatrist, and I said, "I want you to start weaning me off of this stuff." Under her care, we very gradually weaned me off of those things, and now I'm not on anything. I don't take any medication. I used to have panic attacks all the time, but I don't deal with that at all now. I still get situational anxiety, but I realized I was aggravating my mental health. I know there are people that 100% do need medication, but I realized that I was okay without it.

> **NOW, THINGS CAN STILL SUCK, BUT I CAN DEAL WITH THEM BECAUSE RACING FOR RECOVERY TAUGHT ME SO MANY COPING TOOLS.**

Before, I would feel something really strong and really difficult, and I would just shut it down as quickly as possible. I would ignore it and distract myself with food or drinking. Now, I give myself permission to acknowledge, "Wow, I feel kind of like I'm going crazy right now, and I'm really, really anxious." I'll ask myself why I am feeling this way. Am I doing anything right to aggravate that? The beautiful thing about being at Racing for Recovery is they've helped me to flip the script on my anxiety. I'm kind of thankful for it now, because it's this strong reminder that something in my day or in the week overall is out of balance. When my anxiety flares up, nine times out of ten, it means I haven't done something that I normally do to maintain my mental health, or that I'm doing something to aggravate it. Just being able to handle my anxiety without automatically reaching for a Xanax is a self-esteem booster.

The program is definitely goal-based. The ultimate goal is balance, being holistically healthy and balanced. When I've gotten through a difficult issue with Todd, and we've kind of gotten into a lull, he'll say, "Okay, what are we working on next?"

> THERE ISN'T A ONE-SIZE-FITS-ALL APPROACH, WHERE YOU HAVE TO FIT INTO THESE SPECIFIC BOXES. THEY DEFINITELY TAKE WHO YOU ARE AS AN INDIVIDUAL PERSON AND FORMAT AROUND IT, BUT THERE ARE THE COMMON-SENSE LIFESTYLES THAT YOU CAN GO BACK TO.

That's what we can go back to when we're feeling out of balance, to figure out what's missing. I kind of look at it like the roadmap for how to live a balanced life of sobriety.

In the beginning, I had a couple of little cravings to drink. The Super Bowl a couple years ago was the first time I really had a hard time, because a bunch of my friends were there and they were doing shots together, and I kind of felt left out of it. I went into Racing for Recovery the next day, and was sitting in the office talking to Dan, and Todd walked in and asked what was going on. I told him, and that's when he said to me,

> "A FEELING IS JUST A FEELING, YOU DON'T HAVE TO ACT ON IT, AND IT IS GOING TO PASS."

*That was a game changer for me.*

I'm to the point now that I don't want to drink anymore. I just don't have a desire to do it and I know the huge damage it would do to everything I've built in my life. I did a radio interview with Todd a few weeks ago, and on the ride home, he pointed out that because I now have a little bit of public exposure, it's really crucial to not mess up. Now, my sobriety doesn't just affect me and the people immediately around me. I'm an example to other people, and I don't ever want to ruin that for anyone. I love seeing my friends get sober and I really like the people that have become my friends at Racing for Recovery. Watching them do better, hearing their stories, knowing where they were at, seeing where they are now—it's so encouraging. I'm not the only person that struggles with things in life; we all still struggle. Knowing that we're all cognitively present for that struggle now is really cool.

It's amazing that we have this power of choice, but we have to actually choose to get that help, and sometimes people don't get to the bottom of that. Watching some people go back out again, for me, is motivation. I watched that happen to one of my friends that I deeply loved, who was incredibly involved, and went out for six months. He just recently came back. Beautifully, in a recent meeting, he said, "If you think you had guilt and shame walking in here the first time, you have no idea what that is walking in here second time." I try to learn from that. I think about everything that I built up in my life now. I value what I have in my life today. To think about losing that because I made the conscious choice to go back out and drink again is heartbreaking. It's very humbling when that happens, to remember what you have, how blessed you are.

Asking for help and support has been a huge area of growth for me. I've learned that there are people that care about me and that will check in on me, but it's very much my responsibility to stay accountable and to seek that out.

> **PEER SUPPORT IS SUCH A CRITICAL ELEMENT OF SOBRIETY, AND PART OF THAT IS GIVING IT, BUT IT'S RECEIVING IT, TOO.**

I had such a hard time asking for help. It's still something I'm working on. I'm even working on changing the way that I talk about it. I used to have a lot harder time with it, to where I just wouldn't do it. It was paralyzing, because I never want to be a burden to anyone.

When Todd and I started talking about the woman who sexually abused me, I felt like I was dying inside a few times in between our appointments. There were a couple times that I did text him, and then there were a couple times that I let my emotions and my pride get in the way of reaching out. Trust is a really difficult thing for a lot of us, but working up the courage is easier as I'm shown, over and over, that it's safe for me to ask for help. It's hard when you've had decades of trauma to just reverse that mindset. But you ask, you see that the world doesn't fall apart and that it's okay. The next time, it's still paralyzingly scary, but at least you know what the result will be.

> **IT'S REALLY COOL. IT'S SO POSITIVE. PEOPLE DON'T SIT THERE AND SHARE WAR STORIES FROM WHEN THEY WERE USING; THEY TALK ABOUT WHAT THEY'RE STRUGGLING WITH CURRENTLY.**

The philosophy is everybody in that room has done stupid shit, and so we talk about what we're currently struggling with. It's so inclusive. You're hearing from the parents who have lost children—who, by the way, are some of the most dedicated and loving people ever. They're kind of like the moms and dads of the group, which is amazing, because not everybody there has family who will be involved in their lives.

No one from my past has treated me poorly for my change in lifestyle. I'm very fortunate for that, because I know some of my friends have legitimately lost a lot of people; it's been for the better, but it hurts when people walk away from you. I haven't had that experience, but I learned very quickly who was a drinking buddy and who was an actual friend. People that I thought I was so close to for so long, I really wasn't at all. They were just drinking buddies.

We lose people to addiction, whether that's because we have to cut ties, whether people cut ties with us, or because people lose the battle. One of the women who goes to Racing for Recovery just recently lost her son. We acknowledge it. We're also quick to recognize that they made that choice, that it sucks, but they did make that choice. I think in our grief, we try to remember that we're grateful that we're still alive, and we're grateful that we still have breath in our body to be able to make positive choices. We definitely grieve, but I feel like, even with losing people, it's like we treat it like everything else: what can we learn from this and how can we honor their life? The biggest thing that comes to mind for me is the best way that we can honor anyone that lost their battle to addiction is to not lose our lives to addiction and to stay sober. That is an unfortunate part of being in a community where you have people that sometimes don't get the help they need. It's absolutely heartbreaking, and at the same time, it's a really sobering reminder of how short life can be and how thankful we are that we still have the power of choice.

We do a lot of work together, and we do a lot of work on our own, to face ourselves. Songwriting, as far as just working through difficult things, is very therapeutic for me. Whenever I have some negativity going on, I will throw it out into some lyrics, and once it's out there, it's cathartic. I wasn't writing for a really long time. Just recently, in the past few months, I picked it back up. I was so used to writing for it to be a finished product to then crank out for people to hear, so I kind of made the decision when I started writing again that I wasn't going to write with the goal of someone else hearing it, that it was just for me. I think that helps because if I'm the only one hearing it, I don't have to worry about what I'm putting in. If I crank out something that I want to share with people or play at my gigs, that's cool. But I try really hard now to not have that be the goal, so that I can be as vulnerable and as dark as I want to be without somebody being concerned about me.

I put out on my first album in 2017, and all of the songwriting for that album was from high school to right before I released the album. In those lyrics, I hear a lot of loneliness and desperation for love. Some of it's kind of hard for me to listen to, but also it's kind of nice because I'm able to recognize I'm not in that headspace anymore.

My wife and I gig together as a duo at least twice a week; she's the bass player, and I'm on the acoustic guitar. I play three or four other instruments, but that's my main instrument. Then, I'm in another side project, a full band. Since joining Racing for

Recovery, I've learned that playing in a certain area of our town is really stressful for me now. I watch people get hauled off by the cops and people puking in front of me. It's this constant reminder that I don't want to be unhappy like that anymore. We didn't lose out on gigs, we just got a lot more selective. The places that we play at, they're more restaurant-bars. It's an earlier time slot; I used to play until 2:00 in the morning, party with the staff until about 3:30, go get something to eat afterwards, and be home in bed maybe by 6:00 a.m. That life does not appeal to me anymore, so I like the 6:00 p.m. to 9:00 p.m. kind of gig.

My wife is the most supportive person in the entire world. She has come to support group meetings with me, and she's been around the building for special events with me and has gotten to know the people that are important to me from there. She's come in to a couple of my one-on-ones before, which is huge. Shannon is kind of a reserved person, and therapy in general makes her anxious, but even she says Todd makes it incredibly comfortable. When I went vegan, she said, "Let's just make everything in the kitchen vegan," because we both love to cook. She's vegan at home, but she does what she wants out of the house. Even with the drinking, it doesn't bother me to be around her drinking, because she has that off switch. She can have one or two drinks and she's good, and she's very respectful. She doesn't over drink because she knows that would put a lot of stress on me and would just be really hard for me to handle emotionally.

She's been involved in the ways I've wanted her to be from the get-go. She has always told me that she will be as involved as I want her to be.

Some of the things I would tell her, she would need time to process. I don't think it was any surprise to her that there were some things going horribly wrong inside of me; it was so evident out on the physical side, and she was watching me fall apart with panic attacks. There were nights that I was clinging to her for dear life because I felt like I couldn't breathe. I always felt like we communicated really well, but I discovered we didn't really because I wasn't communicating so much. Now, it's really great because I talk to her and let her know when I'm struggling with something, and it feels so much more natural.

The biggest thing that I'm working towards with being sober and getting healthy is that my wife and I want to start a family. We've wanted to since we were in our early twenties, but we were super poor, and there's no way that we could have done it, even if she was the one carrying the baby. I was so overweight, there's no way I could have run after a toddler. I wasn't emotionally healthy enough. My drinking was in the way. To quit drinking and get sober, then get happy with myself, feel good about myself, and get to a point where I felt capable of raising another human being was huge. We actually just started having appointments at a fertility center here. When I have a rough day and I'm having those "you're not good enough" feelings, I can look back two years ago, when I could hardly take care of my pets, let alone myself. Even when you haven't reached the ultimate goals yet, when you're hitting these little milestones, it helps to keep you moving and helps to keep you motivated.

One of my friends who actually just joined the staff at Racing for Recovery has frequently brought her children, and it's made a very positive impact on them, so I definitely want my children involved with it. I want my children to know the mountains that I've climbed and conquered. I think there will be a time and a place for that. I don't want them to be scarred by my scars, but I want them to understand why I am who I am today. I want to inspire them to make positive choices by showing them where my life was and where it is now, that I have the things that I have now because of these positive choices that I've made.

I can't think of a better non-biological family to bring into their lives than the family at Racing for Recovery. It's great because we're there for each other, not just when we're in the meetings, but when we have life stuff happen. People help each other out with rides when they need it, and so it's kind of like that, because I don't have any biological family that lives here, and I don't have the closeness with my mom. It's great because I've gotten to choose those people by being at Racing for Recovery.

The most valuable thing I could tell my younger self would be that you always have the choice to make a good or a bad decision. Every choice that you make has a big impact on your life, even if it doesn't seem like a big one.

> **THE POOR DECISIONS THAT WE MAKE ARE CHOICES, THEY'RE NOT WHO WE ARE. THERE IS ABSOLUTELY NOTHING WRONG WITH WHO YOU ARE. YOU ARE EXACTLY WHO YOU ARE SUPPOSED TO BE, AND YOU NEED TO MAKE THE CHOICES THAT REFLECT THAT.**

I made a series of choices that I wasn't happy with or proud of, and I spent years beating myself up. I've worked so hard to change my mindset, to realize that I did some really awful things, but so has every single person. Some of us have done things that have had a much more profound impact on our lives and caused some really gnarly negative consequences, but at the end of the day, we've all made poor choices.

Learning from those choices and even from my trauma was huge for me, seeing that it caused a lot of problems for me in this area, but because it did, I was able to experience the joy of growth. The fact that I was sexually abused is absolutely horrendous and awful, but if I hadn't gone through that, I wouldn't have certain characteristics that I have today. I wouldn't have gotten out of

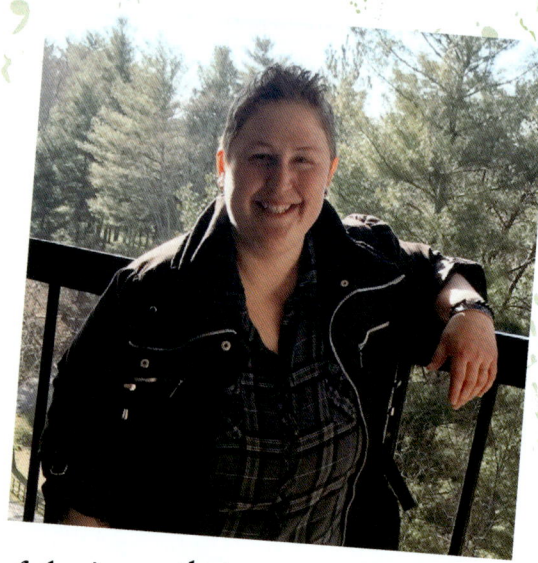

my mom's house, and I probably wouldn't be alive today.

Life just got better. Like I tell my friends now, nothing in my life is perfect in any way, shape, or form by any means, and I still deal with some of the issues that I dealt with before. Things with my mom still aren't good, and I still have life stress, but I can just deal with it now. I'm present for it, which is amazing.

> IT'S KIND OF LIKE NOW, ANYTIME SOMETHING BAD HAPPENS, AND I GET THROUGH IT, AND I HAVEN'T DRANK OR USED ANY KIND OF A DRUG, AND I WAKE UP THE NEXT DAY AND THINGS ARE STILL OKAY—THAT'S A HUGE VICTORY.

That's a self-esteem boosting thing, too. Even though I still struggle with a lot of self-esteem issues, I at least know logically now that those things that I'm thinking in my head are not true. I can feel them, but the feeling does pass.

It's okay that I'm feeling that way, but that's not the actual truth.

I think those voices are always there, kind of in the back of my head, but I'm able to shut them down more quickly, and I know that I can reach out and other people can help me boost my self-esteem. I hope that one day those self-doubts go away, but at least now I'm equipped to deal with it.

I don't call myself an alcoholic. I used to abuse alcohol, but that is not who I am at all. I am a loving person. I'm a good listener. I have had to learn the hard way in the past, but because of that, I'm now a very strong person. I'm intelligent, and I care about people wholeheartedly, and that's who I am. Poor decisions that I made in my life definitely helped to shape me, but me getting drunk and driving up on a curb at night—that's not who I am, that's what I did. It sucks to have to go through all that, but I feel like that's helped me to overcome those things, and even enhanced some aspects of who I am as a person that I definitely did not appreciate before.

Figuring out who you are at your core isn't easy, but some of it is as simple as looking at what you really love. I love to play music. Music is a huge part of my identity. It's at the depths of my soul. It's helped me get through a lot of difficult things. I'm a good musician. I think it's learning what your strengths are and figuring out how to really believe them about yourself. As far as discovering who you are, your identity, that's something that we're all constantly working on. I'm still figuring out things that are really strong, solid characteristics that, six months ago, I didn't know about myself.

You can really not know who you are as a person because you spent so much time numbing yourself out with substances, but I think the jumping off point is knowing that you have value and that you matter. Beyond that, you'll figure out that we're all still growing up. I'm going to continue to figure out what my identity is as a human being, but even on days that I'm questioning what I'm doing and who I am, I know beyond a shadow of a doubt I matter and I have value. Because of that, I have purpose. Even if you don't know what that purpose is, you'll figure that out. The rest of it is part of the journey, and it's okay to not know. That's another huge thing I've learned through all of this sobriety process:

IT'S OKAY TO SAY "I DON'T KNOW."
IT'S TOTALLY OKAY TO NOT KNOW THINGS,
AND THE WORLD WILL NOT FALL APART. I CAN
ALWAYS BE CONFIDENT THAT I HAVE VALUE,
I MATTER, AND I HAVE PURPOSE.
EVERYTHING ELSE WILL WORK ITSELF OUT.

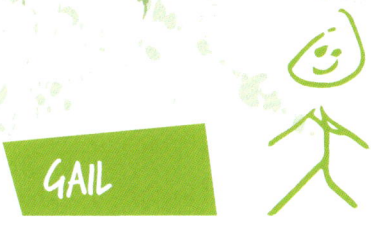

## GAIL

On my birthday in 2015, we learned that my daughter Lauren was doing drugs. A friend of hers texted a family member that Lauren had overdosed and somebody needed to get there right away.

The first time that Lauren overdosed, the ambulance took her to the hospital and she walked away. We went over to her house, my husband and I, and she was still in her hospital gown with all her bandages on. My son came over to support her, and we went home. They ordered pizza, and my son said, "Let's go in the house and clean out all the drugs." Lauren just went off the deep end with him, yelling that she was going to call Children's Services on him and get his kids taken away. It was horrible, and he said, "That's it, you can't threaten my kids," and he walked away.

My husband and I didn't know what was going on. Lauren had a birth defect in her spine; it would shift and pinch her nerves, and it was very painful. They talked about surgery to put rods in and stabilize it, but they were trying to hold off as long as they could. Once you start the surgeries, the weak part just keeps moving up, so you have to have surgery every ten years to put more rods in. She had been prescribed Percocet and various other painkillers for her back and for her endometriosis. She told us that she'd just forgotten how many pain pills she'd taken, and we believed her.

I was diagnosed with breast cancer, so I started right in with surgeries and treatment. The day before I had my mastectomy, my mom died, so I planned her funeral from my hospital room while I was recovering.

Then, Lauren came to us and said she needed help, that she was addicted to drugs. She originally told us it was Xanax. We didn't know what to do, so we were googling recovery centers and where to get her detox. When she went into detox, she told us it wasn't Xanax, it was heroin. The bottom kind of dropped out at that point. She stayed there long enough to detox and then insisted on coming home. If we didn't pick her up, she was going to run away, so we went and picked her up, and she moved home with us. She was arrested shortly after that and put on probation.

I was going through chemo and radiation, still in the thick of my cancer treatment, and nobody was holding Lauren accountable. She would miss probation meetings, she was still using, and she had overdosed several times in my house. It usually happened on a Sunday, when I was watching my granddaughters. At dinner time, we would go up to her room and let her know dinner was ready, and we would find her unresponsive and call 9-1-1. Sometimes we could wake her up, sometimes we couldn't. Sometimes, the EMTs would revive her. Once they made her go to the hospital, once they just let her go home, once we found her and took her to the hospital.

Things got really bad right after Christmas of 2016. Lauren overdosed three times in a couple months. She was arrested again for using drugs and violating probation. She was in jail for two months and then she went to a diversion program here, which was two months as well.

Bruce and I kept it a secret, really until Lauren went to jail. When Lauren went to jail, that's when we kind of opened up. I needed to let people know because she wasn't going to be around for family functions, not as if she went to most of them anyways. But people had seen what she looked like within the past few months, and she didn't look healthy. She looked bad. She lost a ton of weight, she had a lot of scars on her arms from using, her hair was falling out, just all those signs.

I think one of the saddest moments was when we went for our first weekly visit to the diversion program, on Mother's Day. Lauren said, "I'm just a drug addict," and it was like her whole life and soul went out. It was really sad to hear. She was so much more than that.

> MY DAUGHTER SUFFERED FROM ADDICTION. IT'S WHAT SHE DID, BUT IT WASN'T WHO SHE WAS. SHE WAS A VERY GENEROUS, KIND SOUL.

She left all the clothes that she had worn in jail (they had to wear specific grey pants or black pants and a white shirt) for the other girls, because many of them didn't have family members that would help them or even come and visit them. That's the kind of person she was. She would give everything she had to somebody else to make them feel better, even at her own expense. She saw the best, even in drug dealers. She'd tell me things like, "Mom, these aren't bad people." But she couldn't understand that people didn't have to be bad to do bad things to her.

She had been clean for about four months when she was released. I wanted her to go to a halfway house or sober living or something like that, but she came home instead. The first day home, within a couple hours, she put her car into a ditch, so I assumed she probably used as soon as she got out.

We'd promised my granddaughters we'd take them to the spot we always went for family trips in Upper Michigan before school started. So, about a month after Lauren got home, the rest of the family was getting ready for that trip. My son surprised me by calling and saying Lauren could go—that we couldn't live like this forever, and that we had to start putting the pieces back together. It was the first step in trying to make the family whole again. We spent three days up there all together, and she said it was the best time she had ever had in her life.

Lauren had a history of mental issues; she'd been in and out of psych wards since the age of twelve, and she had bad anxiety.

Within two weeks of getting back from our family vacation, I drove her over to Racing for Recovery and parked, because she needed to get some help. Her anxiety was really high, and she said, "Mom, I've got to do this by myself. I'll go, but you gotta let me come over here. You can't force me to do this." I said okay, and she made an appointment for an assessment. She showed up forty-five minutes late, and they had back-to-back appointments. It was a Thursday or a Friday, so they rescheduled her for the following week.

That Sunday, we went up to wake her up for dinner. She was already gone. She had overdosed; her body was cold. My husband and I called 911, and he started doing CPR. EMTs came and worked on her for about an hour and a half, and then she was pronounced dead. **Lauren died on August 27, 2017. She'd only been out of jail for six weeks.**

Monday or Tuesday, my husband and I started planning the funeral. People wanted to donate money, and we wanted it to help other people who were struggling with addictions. So, we went over to Racing for Recovery to see what it was like. It happened to be a Thursday night, when they have their signature meeting. I walked in and talked to Dan. When I told him Lauren had passed away, his face drained of all color. He'd known she was in trouble when she came in late for her assessment, and he'd tried to go after her, but by the time he'd made it outside, she was gone, and she wouldn't pick up the phone. He introduced us to Todd.

We didn't stay for a meeting that week, but we went back the next week, and it just fit. There were other individuals there that had lost kids. I didn't feel like I was alone; somebody else was feeling the exact same way I was, and they were surviving. We've been going there two years now.

Talking with the groups there and all of the kids that have beaten addiction helps me put the pieces together. My husband and I thought we were doing the right things; we wouldn't give her money, for example, but we would go put gas in the car or something like that. Well, she was using that to give drug dealers rides places and things like that in exchange for drugs. If she wanted cigarettes, we'd go buy her cigarettes. I would buy her things like gift cards to McDonald's, so she would have something to eat. I didn't realize that those are things that she would use to buy drugs. I was just so naive about all of this. Lauren would wake me up in the middle of the night and tell me one of her drug dealers was after her and she needed $100 so he wouldn't come to the house. And I believed her because I didn't know any better and I wanted to believe her. I get it now that I enabled her. My husband was probably stronger than I was, but she is my baby girl and part of me was beating myself up over all that: What should I have done differently? What didn't I do? It kind of gave some closure on some things and helped us understand.

There was two years of just sheer hell and not knowing what to do, how to do it, or where to turn. How do you get better if you don't have the right people helping you, a great support system? I was always available for her, but it wasn't what she needed. She needed somebody else that could feel what she was feeling. I wish Lauren would have found Racing for Recovery—I wish she would have made that appointment. I think if she could have seen that group, it would have turned her around. She would have had people to relate to, who knew what she was feeling and what she was going through, people that she could have reached out to and just hung out with that weren't going to go and do drugs. That's what I think pains me the most. If she would have just showed up there on time and talked to Todd and met some of the people that are regulars there, I think we could have had a whole different outcome.

> **RACING FOR RECOVERY HAS HELPED ME FORGIVE MYSELF. SHE DID THIS TO HERSELF; SHE'S THE ONE THAT STUCK THE NEEDLE IN HER ARM.**

She was upstairs in her bedroom overdosing and I was sitting downstairs in my family room. She didn't have to do that. If she was feeling anxious or needed somebody, I was right there, and all she had to do was come and get me. I didn't know what to do, where to go, or how to feel. The range of emotions, everything from anger to fear to terror to pain to sadness and everything in between, all hits at the same time. They helped me accept all of that and say it was okay to feel all those things.

Just being around the other kids that have succeeded brings me hope; although Lauren didn't make it, there are many people who did. Some of the kids at Racing for Recovery have really touched my soul. Jordan was probably the first kid I met there and really talked to, and he gives the best hugs. About two months after Lauren overdosed, Jordan was on the right track, but then he overdosed, and they had to bring him back. His mom goes to the meetings as well. She was talking about how she got the phone call and how everybody from Racing for Recovery just rallied around Jordan after he got out of the hospital, and was there for him, and made sure he was okay. There's Jake and Jeff and so many others. Brittany is a younger girl there, and she is also adopted, like Lauren was, so sometimes the stories she tells, I can identify with more. They fill in the pieces of what Lauren was feeling, what she was going through, how she felt, how horrible the addiction was for her.

There are two individuals at Racing for Recovery that lost kids before Lauren died, Rick and Randy, that are my support system. We bonded over our grief, and we still hurt, but they've really helped me get through it. The moms of those that have beat the addiction are very supportive. We know the isolation of trying to help our children beat this. We know how scary it is to not know where to turn. I very actively expose people I know to where they can get help if they're dealing with this. I contacted several people to tell them to look at Racing for Recovery: "Maybe they can help you figure out what you need, get you assessed, get you into meetings. There are meetings almost every night. I can put you in touch with people who you know you can reach out to at any moment." It's really hard, asking for help. There's a lot of stigma to addiction: what did you, as a parent, do that allowed your kid to get into drugs? We're the typical, middle-class, American family. My husband and I both work, we had three dogs at the time, we had two grandkids. If you looked at us from the surface, you would never think our daughter was addicted to drugs and died from an overdose, but it happens to all walks of life.

> **JUST TELLING PEOPLE THAT THEY AREN'T ALONE, THAT OTHER PEOPLE HAVE GONE THROUGH THIS, AND MOST OF THEM MAKE IT OUT ON THE OTHER SIDE, IS SO IMPORTANT.**

A friend reached out to me to say she'd just found out her daughter was doing heroin and she's in a recovery place. She went to a meeting with me two weeks ago for the first time. She just did not know where to turn or what to do, and she just needed to talk. One of the ladies there brought her a little plaque, just a little gift for her first time being there.

Just the empathy that everybody has is just amazing. You have over a hundred people in these Racing for Recovery meetings and everybody is just a hundred percent behind everybody else. There is no backstabbing or backbiting. Everybody wants you to be successful and beat this and just enjoy life. There's no negativity in there at all; it's very uplifting and calm. We do touch on tough subjects, but you always feel good when you walk away. No matter what kind of day you're having, what kind of week you've had, when you go in there, you get centered again.

Last summer, a friend of mine died of cancer. She was younger than me, and our kids had gone through school together. It was a particularly hard day for me, and Bruce was out of town for a week. I just went onto the Racing for Recovery Facebook site, and I sent a private message. Within ten minutes, somebody responded to me, and said, "Call me up." I never feel like I'm alone, even in the darkest times. Whether it's the middle of the night or early morning, all I have to do is post a private message to Facebook, and somebody will answer me.

A lot of the things that they talk about in those meetings resonate with me as well; I never suffered from drug addiction, but I had anxiety and I was hospitalized for severe depression. When I have a stressful day, I can hear those conversations going on, and it keeps me centered.

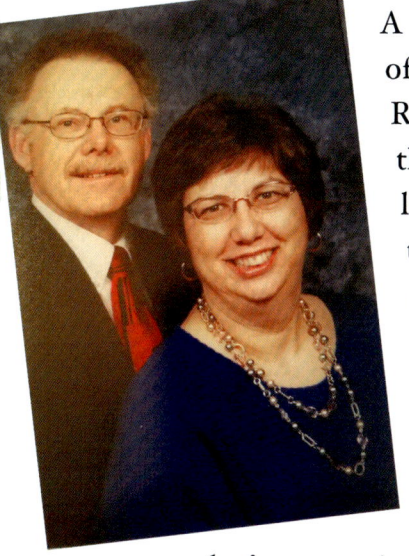

A lot of kids don't have the support of parents, so by going to Racing for Recovery meetings, the kids that are there by themselves can look at us like another set of parents. We try to let them know people do care about them, that they're just not trash that can be thrown out. That's why I geared myself more towards Racing for Recovery than some of the other groups that I've been exposed to since Lauren died. I don't want to just, "Woe is me, my daughter died." It was horrible. Everybody knows that. Like Todd says,

## EVERYBODY KNOWS THE HORROR STORIES—WHAT ARE YOU DOING TO GET OUT OF IT?

I've always been more of an isolated person. I do okay at work or at school or something like that, but when I'm home, I'm a much more of a loner. Even now, I kind of like cocooning and just being in my safe place at home, so sometimes I have to force myself to go to Racing for Recovery meetings. I'll get down, not really depressed, just wondering why anybody would want to hear my story, because Lauren didn't make it. She didn't beat the addiction. I think it's a mental thing that I have to get over, and it doesn't happen all that often, but it does hit. But there's still lessons that Lauren can help me teach others, so they don't have to go down this path. And when somebody else comes in after me, and they have just lost a child or a friend or a relative, I can help them get through that. I just pay it forward. Racing helped me get through it, and now it's my turn to help others get through it, and to let them know that we are here to help. That's beautiful.

Sharing all the stories that I have has helped other people get over their hurdles. My boss' niece was diagnosed three or four months ago with a really aggressive kind of breast cancer. Since I'd been open about my story, he knew he could come to me and bounce things off me. When he was scared, he could talk to me, and I would tell him what she was going to be feeling through her chemo (because she had the same type of chemo that I had), and just some of the things that he could do to help her get through those sixteen awful weeks, when you're sick all the time. I've helped other people handle the stressful situations in their lives better just by being open with mine.

One thing that really opened my eyes up was that when Lauren died, my son's life was in unrelated upheaval. About six weeks later, he got a new job, and things really came around. It hit me in the face like a ton of bricks that life was moving on, there's so much joy, good things were happening, and even though Lauren's not here, I didn't want to miss anything.

I had my life on hold for about two years between the cancer and Lauren, and that's enough. Bruce and I are getting close to retirement age, and I want to enjoy that time. I will always honor Lauren. I will always remember her. She was my other half. We did everything together. It was really hard losing my mom and my daughter, the two people closest to me. There's a big emptiness there. I couldn't go talk to my mom about what Lauren is going through. Lauren wasn't there to go with me to see movies or go out shopping and that sort of stuff, so there's a big emptiness there, but as my granddaughters are getting older, I can share more of those experiences with them.

This morning, I picked my granddaughter, who's nine, up for daycare, and she was just running late, and I made a conscious choice not to be upset. I sat and watched the birds playing in the trees and just let her do what she needed to do in the time frame she needed. It wasn't going to do me any good, being upset with her, and it certainly wasn't going to do her any good. Can't find your socks? We'll go to Walmart and buy you a pair of socks, not a big deal. It's all in how you choose to handle situations, and I try to do it on a more positive note. That's what I try with the people that work for me and with friends and neighbors. I try to stay on the positive side, and I think Racing for Recovery has helped solidify that.

I don't want to waste my life being stuck. It'd be really easy for me to play into the "Woe is me, why does all this bad stuff happen to me that I can't control" mindset. My daughter died. My mother died. I've gone through thirteen surgeries with my cancer. I could play all these cards, but that keeps me stuck. That's not who I am. That's part of my history, my life, but it's not who I am, and I don't really want to be identified like that.

One of Lauren's friends contacted me months after she died and told me that he was the one that first gave her heroin; she'd had really bad anxiety, and he told her that he had something that would help her with that. He said he wished it was him that died, not Lauren. And part of me was like, "Yeah, I wish it was too," but then I realized that wasn't true. She's in a better place. Her and my mom had a really close relationship, so I'm sure they're up there together, bugging my dad. What happened to Lauren was horrible, but I don't want anybody else to die in place of her. I don't want anyone to overdose, ever.

So, I wrote this piece about the last two hours of Lauren's life, from the moment we found her until the coroner took her away, because I think it could help someone. The first time Lauren overdosed, she said, "I know it's scary to see me do this, but all you've got to do is throw ice water on my face, knock me around." People struggling with addiction minimize the possibility of dying, but it happens—and it doesn't have to.

An Open Letter to those battling addiction, from a mother...

> *To those of you in an addiction, I wanted to reach out to you and share my story. I wanted you to see what this is like from the other side of the addiction, from someone who loves you, cares about you, would give their life for you....*
>
> *The last day of my daughter's life—August 27, 2017.*
>
> *It was a normal day—chatting, running errands, enjoying a Sunday. Around 4:00 pm, she came bopping in the front door. I was starting dinner. We exchanged some pleasantries and she went to her bedroom. Around about 5-ish, my husband came in from a bike ride. He checked on things, then went upstairs to change his clothes for dinner. I asked him to let Lauren know that dinner was almost ready.*
>
> *Things dramatically changed in that instant.*
>
> *He yelled to me that Lauren was unresponsive. I called 911 as I was running up the stairs to get to my beautiful daughter. I had 911 on speaker phone as my husband and I lifted her off the bed to get her on a solid surface to start performing CPR.*

She was ashen, her body limp. The memory burned into me is that her body was chilly to the touch. CPR was started, I could hear Bruce counting the compressions as I raced down the stairs to let in the emergency medics. Little did I know that was the last time I would ever see my daughter.

The medics arrived, along with the police, sheriff and everyone else – they went to her bedroom. They relieved Bruce from CPR, and started compressions, hooked her up to machinery and started breathing for her. Once the medics arrived, I was no longer allowed upstairs—partly because there was little room in a bedroom for the life-saving events that were occurring and partly because if the worst happened, they didn't want me witnessing the horror of it all. An officer stood by the bottom of the steps keeping me at bay. I wanted to get to her, I was afraid to get to her—time stood still.

I remember asking the officer as I heard the beeps of the EKG if that was her heartbeat—he said it was. My heart screamed with joy—we got her back. But that wasn't the case. The beeps were from the chest compressions. I couldn't move, I couldn't stand still. I was in shock. I paced in and out of the house. The street was lined with emergency vehicles. Some neighbors stopped by. Some stayed, some tried to offer comfort, some watched in horror not being able to turn away.

I remember saying that I thought that she was gone—that

*we lost her. I couldn't cry—I wanted this to be a bad dream. I called our son—he asked what he should do, if he should come over. There was nothing he could do, and the last memory of her that I wanted for him was a recent vacation that we had with the entire family a few short weeks earlier.*

*Bruce came down intermittently during this time, they were working on her, but it wasn't good. We called family members—the screams of anguish that I heard from them are forever resounding in my soul.*

*Then it was over, the paramedics came down, they had worked on her for an hour with no response. It was time to let her go peacefully. It was 6:40 pm. The paramedics left, one officer stayed, they contacted the coroner's office. They took our stories individually—as to what occurred. A few family members had shown up by then, hugging us, not knowing what to say. It was all a horrible dream—it just had to be.*

*I couldn't be at the house when the coroner took her away, I walked the neighborhood, but saw the vehicle drive by with her lifeless body inside. My beautiful daughter had lost her battle with the demons.*

*My best friend was gone—who would be bopping in and out of the house, who would be texting me, who would be meeting me for lunches, who would watch TV with me*

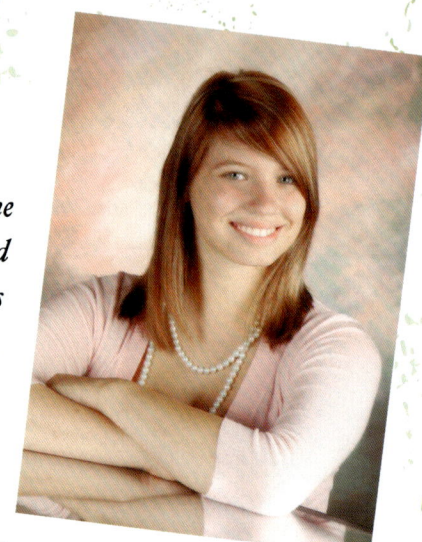

*laughing at how horrible some wedding dresses looked. Who would let me tease her, who would laugh as I told her she had a round little face, who would look forward to trips to Mackinac Island. Who would be my daughter?*

*She was 24 years old. She had been using for a couple of years. She had gone through detox. She had spent time in jail, and CAD and come out clean and healthy looking a month before. But the drug called to her. She answered that call. And the drug won.*

*Did she realize, when she came home that afternoon and went upstairs with the intention of using, that it would be her last act? No more chocolate malts, no more sunsets, no more smelling the sweet smell of spring, no more watching her nieces laugh and play and grow up, no more dreams. No more tomorrows...*

*I beg all of you who are reading this, to realize how this affects everyone around you. This happened to my daughter, but it could have been anyone. Please get help, get support, talk to people, scream at the top of your lungs that you need help, stop using—it is too big to go at it alone.*

*The addiction can kill you. There may not always be a tomorrow. You cannot always assume it will be someone else. And it could be your mom finding you, or your dad, your little brother or sister, son, daughter or spouse. And that is the memory that will be etched forever in their soul.*

*Please—you are the only one that can quit your addiction. I beg of you.*

*The Mother of Lauren Elizabeth*

*Mar 2, 1993 – Aug 27, 2017*

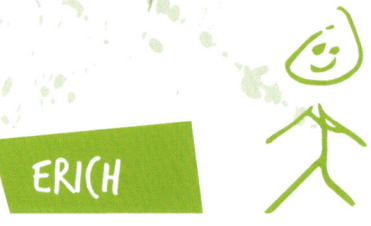

My birth father abandoned me before I was born, so I never met the guy. He was a hardcore alcoholic. He could have been a very successful baseball player, I was told, but alcohol was too much a part of his life.

My stepfather came into my life when I was about four. He was very much a workaholic. He was very good about putting food on the table, but he was pretty much absent emotionally. I don't know if it would have been regarded as abusive back then, but it hurt me badly, emotionally and mentally. From a very young age, I never felt as though I measured up or was worthy in his eyes. I remember getting in a fight with the neighbor boys. He went out and threw rocks at them, basically, and told them that he had to stick up for me because I wasn't capable of doing it myself. Even the memory of that still hurts.

My mother was always very supportive, but it wasn't really her approval I was seeking; it was Dad's. He didn't praise frequently; when he did it, he meant it, and it did count, but I always needed more. We have a much better relationship now than we've ever had. The way that his behavior affected me broke his heart; he didn't mean to hurt me. He's just human. Back then, though there was just a lot of wanting to please him, and wanting to be something that maybe I wasn't. When I look back on it now, it's kind of new for me to realize some of the ways that I felt, and some of the reasons that I felt that way.

Dad tried to be my baseball coach for a while when I was twelve or thirteen, and ended up never showing up for that. Someone else ended up taking over. In my early teens, my mom and dad separated once, and then they got divorced, so I saw even less of him.

My dad actually gave me a beer on the way back from a softball tournament when I was about seven years old, and I think I drank most of it. My first experience being really drunk was freshman year of high school. Some neighbor kids and I got together, and we all passed out and had to be dragged to our respective houses. My dad literally dragged me up the back steps—there were many—and I woke up the next morning having to go to a varsity wrestling meet. I threw up all over the high school. It was a bad, bad day and I didn't touch it again for a couple of years.

As I started to reach that age where girls were very important, alcohol, in my perception, helped me fit in. I never really felt like I fit in anywhere, but drinking helped me open up. It made me feel like one of the gang, because everybody else was doing it, so I was accepted and loved, I thought. It was very popular where I grew up. On Friday night, you would go to the football game, drink and hang out. We smoked a little pot here and there, but for the most part, it was just drinking.

I was about eighteen when it became a regular thing. I went to school at Kent State University, but I never graduated. I had more friends that liked to drink there, and I did that a lot, instead of going to class and doing other things. It was more fun and less scary for me to just drink with my buddies, and my grades reflected that. I got a job waiting tables, bartending, working the restaurant scene, and after work, we would go and drink.

Along the way, I began to feel a sense of failure because I was not living up to my potential. When I did apply myself, I got very good grades. I tested very highly, and I think in my mom's and dad's eyes, I was going to be the doctor in the family someday. It was not happening at this point, and I could always sense some disappointment from both of them. That played into me beginning to create my own false world. I would tell lies about scenarios, when I didn't live up to this standard that I thought was perfection. I lied a lot to cover my drinking, how I spent money, or to make me feel better about myself. I would try to make myself feel better and heal some kind of self-esteem. It was one of my biggest problems. I was always measuring and trying to validate myself according to other people's opinions of me. I didn't know what I wanted. I was too afraid to pursue anything, because if I wasn't going to be perfect at it (and I hadn't found that thing that I could be perfect at), it wasn't worth pursuing. If I was going to fail, I was just going to create another lie to cover my perceived failure of not being perfect.

I moved to North Carolina when I was twenty-three. All I'd been doing was drinking and bartending and getting into one bad relationship after another. My mom understandably kind of threw her hands up, and told my dad, "I don't know what to do with him anymore—he needs you in his life." So, my dad helped me get a job at the injection molding company he worked for, and I picked up and moved there to be with him.

I was pretty decent at this job, and I moved up rapidly. I started competing with Dad along the way. I didn't enjoy it. I didn't like doing automotive or plastics engineering. I just wanted to do it because I thought it would earn his approval, and, frankly, I just wanted to be better than he was at it.

Over the three years we worked together, I got to know my dad. We opened up to each other a lot, but I still kind of kept those things that hurt from the past to myself unless I was really drunk. Then I would bring them up, but neither of us would remember it later. There was never any resolution to it. We would go to this little bar in Burlington, North Carolina, called The Bedrock, all the time, and we drank and chased women. All we did was work and then go drink, which fit in perfectly with the automotive injection-molding world. You'd put in a lot of hours, and needed to go drink afterwards.

I was constantly pushing the envelope because of the crowd I surrounded myself with. I never consciously pursued the thought that I might have a problem, even though drinking was really all I wanted to do. I would work for the money to go out and drink, so nothing was getting interrupted, but even my friends would kind of look at me like, "Wow, he drinks a lot," which I did. I did not drink for pleasure. I drank to escape and to hope that somebody would buy whatever lies I was going to tell them in hopes they would accept me.

This went on for about three years, until my dad decided one day, out of the blue (that's kind of his nature), that he was getting remarried and moving a couple hours away. After he left, I had free rein to basically do whatever, and my drinking really took off. I kept on that same path of 'work hard, play hard, and drink more.' It progressively got worse. Basically, from 1999 or 2000 to 2007, I drank every day.

I was unhappy. I hated my job. I made good money, but I didn't pay my bills like I should have. I had a car repossessed. Towards the end, people were just through with me because they knew all I really wanted to do was drink, and that was going to take priority, that was the thing my life revolved around. If there was an activity outside of the norm that didn't involve drinking or I couldn't drink while I was there, that was a problem.

I had some enablers around me at work. Since I was good at my job, they would look the other way, but I would drink before work just so I wouldn't shake badly enough that I couldn't write my name. I would drink at work, out in my car during breaks. I would drink after work, and then, on the weekends, it was time to just party at bars with my so-called friends. I got multiple DUIs in the midst of this—I have a total of four, none since 2009. It caused me more trouble, but it was still never enough to make me quit.

I moved back to Ohio and started a pretty good relationship, one that would have been very healthy if I could have been healthy. It's one that I'm actually trying to recover now. We were together for many years. Those were the first times I'd tried to become sober. I went through the Salvation Army, where it's a lot of religious practice. I did learn a few things there, but at no point did anybody ever ask the questions, "Why do you drink? What is it that has gotten you drinking? What is it that's perpetuated this drinking?" No one tried to get to the bottom of what I was running from.

I managed to stay sober for a little under three years, I think, but I was miserable. I hated what I was doing. I hadn't faced any of the demons that I still had. I was just not drinking. That was the only thing that I was doing. I finally left the automotive world after a drinking episode got me a charge of communicating a threat to one of my fellow co-workers. I got thrown in jail for thirty days. They locked the plant down; it was not a good scene. They thought I was going to come in and shoot the place up, but

I didn't have a gun. That was not my intent, but it was the post 9-11 thing, where any kind of threat of physical violence could be taken to a pretty high level. That nearly ended my relationship. You would think that would be enough for me to get sober.

What finally happened was that all my lies started getting exposed, and it just had these major ramifications. I love my significant other, and I love her daughter—I always thought of them as my wife and my daughter. The whole time, though, I was lying to them about things that were ridiculous; just these stupid lies, not an attempt to hurt anybody else, but to make me look better. A lot of deception went on, both with money, and other things. My significant other would take medication for pain. I took some of her medication at points and I would try to convince her that she had miscounted or things like that, so I was gaslighting her. When she found out about some of my lies, she was so incredibly hurt. I finally realized what bad choices I'd been making, and I knew I had to change. It was the path that led me here to Racing for Recovery.

I'd been living in the hotel right across the street from Racing for Recovery as part of a detox program, but the only way to get into Racing for Recovery was to have Medicaid Ohio. The detox was supposed to arrange that for me, but it didn't get done. My two weeks were up, and I was going to be out on the streets at the end of the day.

I ended up walking downtown to Toledo to sit at the job and family services place, just praying that I could get this Medicaid done in one day's time. That just doesn't happen, but I sat there, and I waited, and I talked to as many people as I could. I figured they were going to kick me out, but they didn't. I said, "I really need to be at Racing for Recovery, and I need to be able to stay there. I don't have a place to live. I'm homeless. I have nothing." I guess I talked to the right people, because they got my Medicaid pushed through that day.

So, I walked back from downtown Toledo—it was about ten miles—to Racing for Recovery and talked to Dan. He stood there, looking at this piece of paper that I gave him in disbelief: "You got this today? Wow, man, that doesn't happen." As I'm sitting out in the common area, Todd Crandell, who I'd never met before, walks out and says, "Which one of you just walked from here to downtown to get Medicaid to get in our program and walked back?" Then he told me, "That's what I want out of people, that kind of desire. That's what I want here." He made it clear to me that I had a value, that I mattered.

Rachel told me,

> **"YOU KNOW WHAT? EVEN IF YOU DON'T LOVE YOU, YOU'RE GOING TO LEARN TO, AND WE WILL LOVE YOU UNTIL YOU FIGURE IT OUT."**

They lived up to that in every way, shape, and form. I've never been around something like this but they said right up front, "Let's restart this. Let's face the demon. Let's get to what hurts, why it hurts, the trouble you've been through, and sort this out. Let's help you to understand that you have value, that you can do this, and that it is possible you don't ever have to drink again."

It was my introduction to reality in my new world. The fact that Todd sat there and never judged made me feel like he got me. He could relate things through his own experiences and some of the things that he had been through, and that really, really helped. At that point, I knew I could kind of leave the outside out there, devote myself full-time to me in here, and do what I really, really needed to do and get better, not just stop drinking. It had to be everything. I had to heal. I had to get stronger about how I felt about me, to get to know me, to reestablish and reexamine my values—what do I believe, what trips my triggers, what are the things that I'm afraid of, what am I running from, how do I not be afraid of them, how do they not rule my life?

> YOU HAVE A GROUP OF PEOPLE IN HERE, SOME OF THE GREATEST PEOPLE I COULD EVER HOPE TO GO THROUGH THIS WITH, AND WE ARE TRYING TO FIND THE SAME ANSWERS, AND WE SHARE THEM WITH EACH OTHER.

Over the course of this last year, I've gotten a lot of answers. I know they'll keep coming, and there'll be a lot of work to put in. It was exactly what I needed to realize I was good enough. Maybe I hadn't found my niche or what I was going to do for the rest of my life, maybe I hadn't found me, but after that first conversation with Todd, where I told him how I felt about me and my shortcomings, it felt like the weight of the world had been lifted off my shoulders. I have established now that I don't have limits anymore. As I got these small victories under my belt, honestly being who I was, and not having to be somebody else or feeling compelled to be somebody else, I began to know that I am good enough, that I don't have the limits that I thought I had, and that I'm not going to be perfect.

One of the best things that I do every day is I go into the weight room with the goal to fail. I want to fail every single time I walk in there, and it takes a lot of that fear away. I want to keep going. I want to do my workout, press my body and my mind as far as I can. The other thing is there's no instant gratification with working out, lifting weights, and training; it comes over time. You can see the results, but you have to be patient for them. It's helped me with patience, and knowing that I can push myself over all these perceived obstacles.

When you get down in the arena, there's a lot of people that sit around and watch and want to criticize. When you get into that arena, you're going to get your ass kicked; it's just what happens. Along the way come victories, learning about what makes me able to stay in the arena, and it's something I can be proud of. But, I have to adhere to those basic things—the drive, the work, the honesty, knowing when I need help, knowing when I need to talk to somebody, when things aren't going well.

A lot of it was just trying and pushing day by day and realizing that failure wasn't killing me. I had this realization that the people who were chewing the dirt around me were the ones that were important to what I was trying to do. In their eyes, failure wasn't making me less of a person because they were doing it right alongside me. The critic's opinion of me is not important until they get down in the arena with me.

It was so comforting to know that I was not alone in here. So many of the people that I look up to have been through this, and they had the same fears, the same doubts about themselves. If I would have walked in these doors and talked to these people, I would have never believed that they struggled with some of the things that I did. To find out that they have and see where they are now, what they do now, who they are—well, the proof is in the pudding. It's that substance. I spent some time with Todd, and I realized he's normal—and I say that in the most loving way. He's not on some pedestal, he's a guy with dedication who gives everything he does everything he's got. If he can do this, I can do this, and it brings so much reality to it.

When I started, it was about getting the demons out of the dark and cleaning house. I then realized that what was left was still a structure that I could build on, and I'd never had that before. I've never felt in my life a confidence that was real. I have the ability now to trust myself, I can trust my actions, and I can believe that I'm not going to let myself down. And it's weird to have that real solid feeling anytime, probably from numbing myself throughout the years. I don't think I ever had the benefit of gaining that wall of toughness people build through facing adversity, through facing obstacles that a "normal" or "well-adjusted" person would go through, and build that belief in themselves. It was totally foreign territory to me, and instead of feeling that uncomfortable feeling, that pain, that sense of this could go either way, I might win or lose, instead of facing up to it, doing it, and getting past it, I would always run, so I didn't know what it felt like to be "tough" and do what was best for me. It was easier to run, but now any challenge that comes up for me brings a little bit of a smile on my face. I think, "You know what, yeah, let's do this, let's see what we can and can't do," and if I fail, I'll get up, I'll try again, but at no point am I going to reach for the bottle, at no point am I going to bring that back into my life or make up a lie. I'll just tell you I didn't get it done, but I'm going to keep doing it until I do.

Something huge I picked up that'll stay with me for the rest of my life, is

> **I WANT TO SET GOALS SO HIGH THAT I CAN'T REACH THEM, BUT I CAN GROW INTO THE PERSON WHO CAN REACH THEM.**

It's not the treasure at the end of the rainbow, it's becoming the kind of person that can build that kind of life to reach that. It's more the journey. When Todd took me to the IRONMAN in Maine, I got to see these amazing people push themselves beyond the limits of what I thought was possible. I saw people of all age groups, all disabilities, doing some of the most amazing things I've ever seen people do. It made me understand that the body will react with pain and react in whatever way it wants, but your mind can make you do whatever you tell it to do. You are in control of that. If you have that kind of desire, you're going to take the pain to do it. If you just look at the obstacles as surmountable, victory may not come overnight, but it'll happen if you continue to push it to happen.

One of the things I never knew is that what was once our biggest weakness will someday be our greatest strength. I firmly believe that it's okay that what you see from me is what you get. I don't typically use a lot of words. I'm usually considered one of the

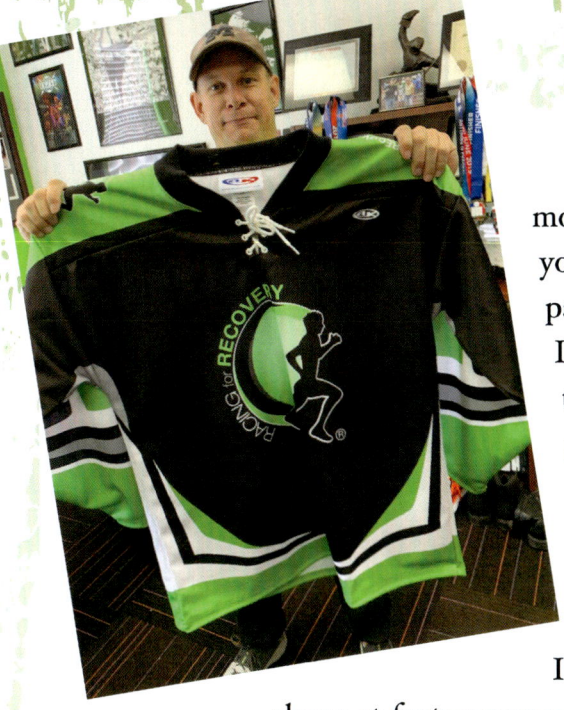

more quiet people here. If you walk with me down my path every day, and see what I do, you'll see everything that I'm about. I'm a person now that likes to explore the extent of my capabilities in every way that I can, scholastically and physically especially. I love to push. I'm in better shape at forty-seven years old, and my health has improved drastically. I watch what I eat. I watch how I conduct myself around others to try to be the real person that I am inside. I'm caring, I'm kind, I'm pretty funny, I'm reasonably intelligent, and I'm loyal to a fault. I am always supportive of those who want better, and I want so badly for everyone that walks through these doors to know that they are of value, that they can reach heights that they never imagined.

I started getting to the root cause of what scared me and why I had such little belief in my own capabilities. Why I was always trying to validate myself with other people. What my values were. What I wanted to be. What I wanted to do.

Life has been amazing. I'm starting to get connections back.

I'm starting to get that trust back. Again, it's not been through words—they could give a damn about my words, and for good reason. I gave them the foundation for 95% of what they thought of me, so I can't blame anybody for what they might feel. I've had to sit back on many occasions, and there will be many more to come, to listen to the ways that I've hurt them with what I've done, but I'll do that if it means that I may get a chance to have them back in my life. That guy who I was is not going to be there again, and I'll take the beatings as they come because it's worth it. That's the other thing that I know scares a lot of people in here, that they don't know what's on the other side. I can assure you it's good, whatever it is. It may not be what you expected, but it's good.

There are times when I get anxious in a situation. If I get really anxious, I will, in the back of my mind (that old spot), create a scenario to get me out of it. I literally have to consciously pause sometimes and go okay, here's the truth. I was a liar so long, it became second nature, so that's something I check myself on. It is much, much easier now to tell the truth, and much more instant. The worst thing that can happen to me if I tell the truth is still not even close to the worst thing that could happen if I lie.

My values were much the same when I was younger as they are now, but I betrayed them all by trying to become someone else who I thought was going to be accepted. I would be whoever was popular, whatever made me cool, even if that betrayed my own values, simply to feel loved or accepted. Now, I really don't give what you think about me, what I am, or who I am; funny enough, that's probably earned me better friends and better relationships than I ever had. I'm not scared of having to back up a lie or trying to figure out where I left off with this lie with this person. It's just so much simpler, and it's so much easier to follow.

I'm working so hard right now to rebuild relationships with some key members of my family that make me very happy. I'm around my mother a lot more, around my niece and nephew, who love to hang out with me now instead of being the absentee uncle they were used to.

I would love to see my significant other again, but I recognize she's got to heal, too. That'll be done on her timeline, if she wants it to happen at all. I want her in my life very much because of who she is and what she means to me, but even if she decides that's not going to happen, I'm going to be okay. I don't want a relationship that she feels obligated to be in. I want her to want to be with who I am. I like to think she does and that's the only reason we're still texting, but I hurt her badly. I tried to imagine what it must look like from her perspective, all of the questions that run through her brain: Why didn't I trust her enough to tell the truth? Why didn't I love her enough to tell her the truth? The only thing that's going to reinforce me being true and who

I truly am is action. I consistently want to be who I am, not something to try to make her like me better, because that's just not going to work. It's got to be me.

I try to let other people notice the changes I make, and not say "Hey, look what I'm doing." That feels more real to me, because I know what I'm capable of building up in my own head. I would rather it just be evident to other people.

Never before in my life was I able to bench press over 300 pounds. That was always something I wanted to do, and I'd lied about doing it. I actually got video of me doing it now, the real thing, at age forty-seven. The very first race that I ever ran in my life was a 10k, and my mom and my sister and everybody asked, "Are you sure?" I said, "I'm going to do this, and I'm going to finish it." I think when I did, they all kind of said, "I think he's sticking around. This might actually be real." That's what I want to continue to do, I want the changes I'm making to come from my actions, not from what I can tell you I'm doing. Words can be flowery, and I've used them way too much in my life. I want there to be substance to everything I do.

I'm never going to go back into the jobs that I had before. Over the course of the last year, I figured out what I want to do. I recently got my CDCA, my license to be a chemical dependency counselor's assistant. I am also about to take a personal training certification exam for Ohio, so I'm doing things that are close to me, that I love. I may not be a millionaire, but it is the things I wanted to do before but didn't because I was afraid I would fail or other people wouldn't be impressed by. I know now that if I'm happy with who I am, other people can beat it. There's a lot that's changed in just a year's time, but it's only beginning.

I don't want to just exist, but to live, to be happy, to push myself to new limits. Crandell embodies all of that. When he got sober and decided he was going to do an IRONMAN, he didn't even know how to swim. He just set this goal, and he's been doing it ever since. I realize that I can put as much effort into making myself better in all these areas of my life as I did to destroying myself, and that's what I want to do.

My worst day in this lifestyle is better than my best day drunk; I can't imagine doing it again. I don't have an urge to run away anymore. People ask me, "Did you get over your anger, your fear, your trauma?" I think of it like that cartoon high-voltage switch. A year ago today, if they flipped that switch, it would be enough to send me off into a tailspin, go drink, and just destroy everything that I had done. At that point, it was just one flip of the switch, if they knew how to do it.

I can still see that switch on the wall, but there's no current running to it. You can flip that thing all day long, you can do whatever you want, and I can see you flipping that switch, it just does not drive me to fear anymore. I don't have a fear of anything that I face. I've lost loved ones, my family, my grandfather died, but at no point did I think about drinking or hiding. There were people drinking around, and I felt, at that point, I needed to be there for my family. I needed to be there to help these people while they're hurting, because I am capable.

I've worked too hard on me to give this up. Now, I like who I am, and I'm getting to the point where I love it. It's going to take some time, but it's turned 180 degrees and I don't want to drink anymore. I don't care who flips that switch. There's no more power there.

My problem wasn't the alcohol. The alcohol was the gun I was going to use to finish the job. I was killing myself by my behaviors, my beliefs, my inability to be in love with who I am, and when I got to the root of that, and start fixing that and building that back up, I realized I don't need the substance anymore. It was doing something for me that I could have been doing for myself the whole time.

> **THERE IS NO SUCH THING AS RELAPSE. IT'S A CHOICE. YOU HAVE A CHOICE WHETHER YOU WANT TO GO BACK.**

I used the idea it was a disease as a huge crutch. Okay, maybe I had a predisposition for addiction, but alcohol is an inanimate object. I put it in my own hand, and I put it in my own mouth, so I have the choice to stop that at any time that I want to. If I'm stuck on a desert island with a diabetic, you don't give me alcohol and don't give him insulin, one of us is going to die, and it ain't me. That choice not to drink is empowerment.

> **WE CAN TAKE THOSE THINGS THAT ARE HURTING INSIDE US, ALL THAT PAIN, THEN TRANSFORM IT INTO OUR GREATEST STRENGTHS.**

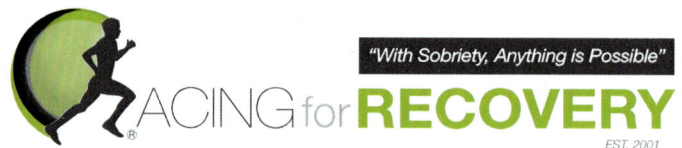

"With Sobriety, Anything is Possible"

ACING for RECOVERY

EST. 2001

## AFTERWORD

On July 28, 2019, I stood on the beach in Delaware, Ohio for my 48th IRONMAN 70.3 event. To some, that may seem like an impossibly big number—to me, it illustrates PERSEVERANCE, along with the Racing for Recovery slogan **WITH SOBRIETY ANYTHING IS POSSIBLE.** I love doing IRONMAN for my health, to travel and meet new people and experience different cultures, and, of course, to achieve goals. Most importantly, though, I participate in IRONMAN events to promote Racing for Recovery along the way, so others may find their "IRONMAN" in whatever passion they pursue. Sobriety is not all about IRONMAN, but it sure is living life to the fullest through a balanced holistic lifestyle.

I could not be in a better place right now. My family is healthy and happy, I have sobriety and inner peace, and Racing for Recovery employs fifteen awesome people and is growing and helping more people every day. Two of our success stories, Andy and Chris, were standing with me on that beach, getting ready to do their first IRONMAN 70.3 race, and several Racing for Recovery peers were on hand to support them.

As I looked at the beautiful sunrise, I reflected back. A year ago, on that same beach, I was preparing to do the same race when Andy told me that next year, he was doing it with me. I also met Mari, who approached me to share her story of losing her brother-in-law to alcohol and suicide. She told me that Racing for Recovery and my books have helped her tremendously. My heart glowed. That's why I was out there on the beach one year ago, and that's why I was back out on that beach today.

When I started Racing for Recovery in 2001, all I wanted to do was make the kind of impact on people that Andy and Mari have felt. I had a vision of showing everyone affected by addiction and self-destructive behaviors that recovery is possible, you can achieve anything you desire, and you never have to use drugs and alcohol again. If I shut the doors at Racing for Recovery today (which I won't), I could say I achieved my goals.

But my life's purpose was, is, and will continue to be reaching more and more people.

That's where this book comes in. That's where you come in. The opportunity to help you is not a burden—it is an incredible, incredible gift. Thank you.

I wish you peace and motivation as you carry on in your journey of self-betterment.

TODD CRANDELL

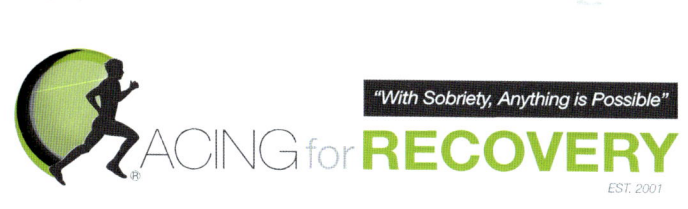

"With Sobriety, Anything is Possible"

RACING for RECOVERY

EST. 2001

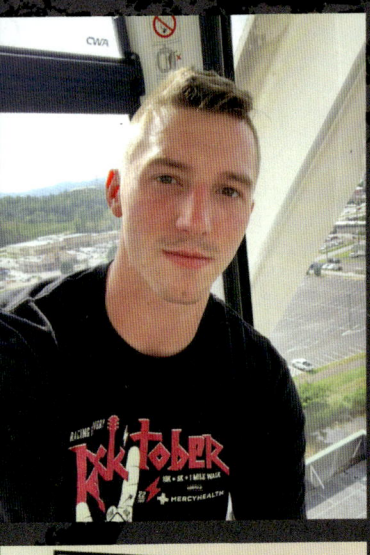

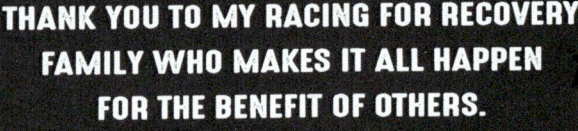

THANK YOU TO MY RACING FOR RECOVERY
FAMILY WHO MAKES IT ALL HAPPEN
FOR THE BENEFIT OF OTHERS.

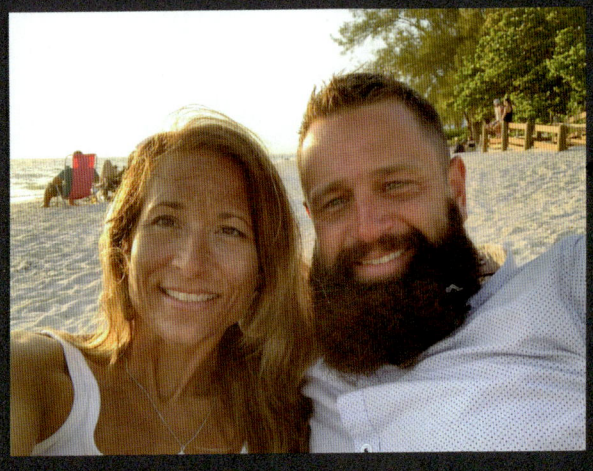

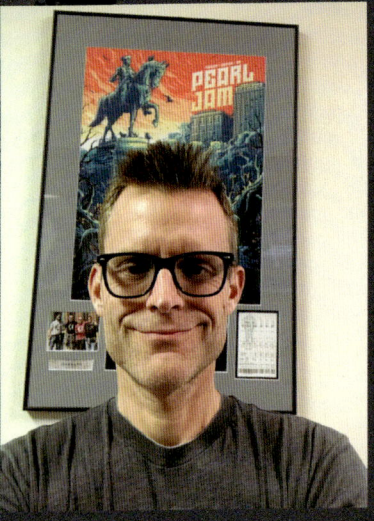

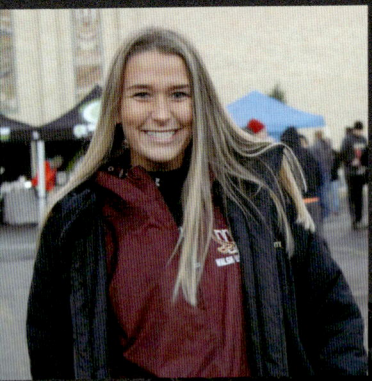

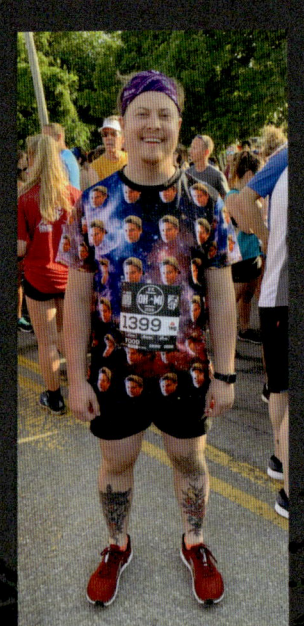

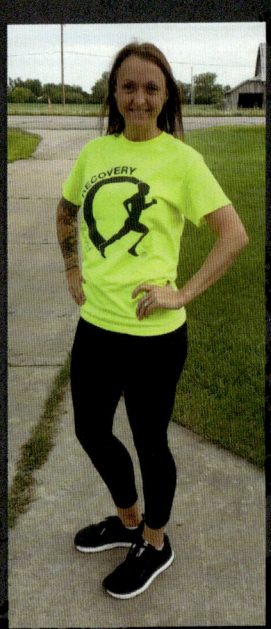

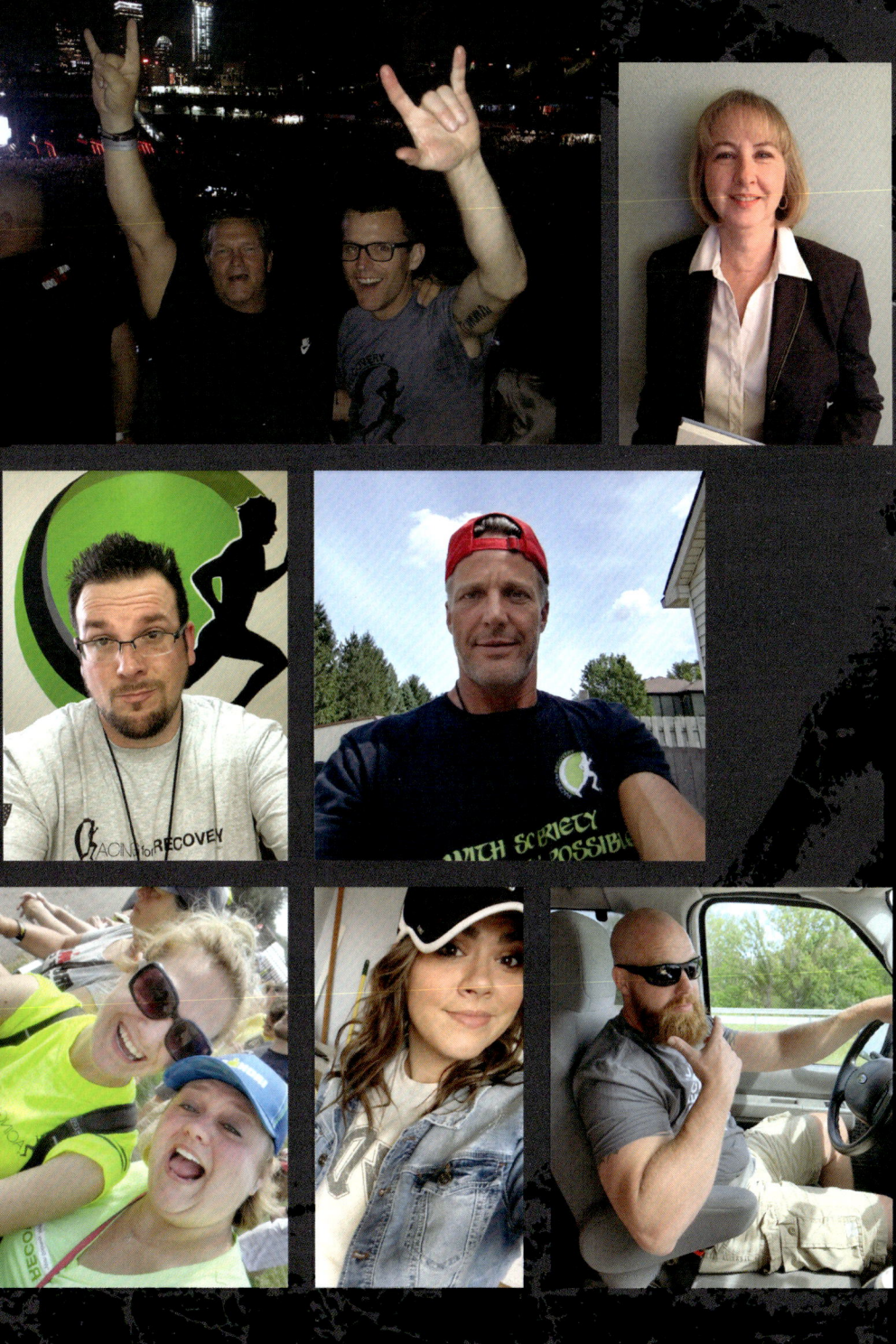

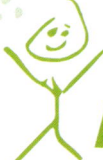

Brendon A Ingram Gave me hope which turned to self value which turned to purpose which turned into the me I am and the future I have again #forevergratful

---

Alvarez Lazlo Racing For Recovery taught me that there is more to recovery than just remaining sober. I've learned to love myself and to actually live life and not just exist. I trust myself again and know my self worth! Drugs are not an option in this beautiful beautiful life I am living today! Thank you Racing For Recovery! ❤️

---

Kimberly M Sheppard It's help me learn that drinking is a choice not a disease. 💚 Helped me cope with my sons passing. Thank you Todd.

---

Andy Nunley Racing for Recovery gave me an opportunity for me to put in the work to improve my life. With continuous support and guidance through one of the hardest thing i ever had to deal with.... figuring out why I kept giving up on myself and learning to cope with those self destructive thoughts by building self esteem and confidence through healthy activities. Im forever grateful for that. Also i got a boatload of awesome friends now too. 😀

---

Lisa Meyer In BRUTAL brevity:
1.education & support to get sober led to
2.improved self-esteem
(a-quitting drinking was one less reason to feel horrible about self
b-unconditional compassion)
3.led to healthier choices
a-like the courage to find out how bad my spine was, & to get it fixed led to
4.sense of efficacy & less pain led to
5.confidence to apply for a life-changing tho temporary job which led to
6.desire for- & sense of worth of- a better life which led to
7.3mos treatment for eating disorders that the alcohol was covering up led to
8.being slightly okay with not knowing

---

Julie Werner Bauknecht It has brought me back my nephew

Julie Brinkman Racing for recovery helped restore our family by teaching our son how to live and love his sober life.

Stan Nowicki And help me work on every area of my life just not being alcohol and drug free

Amanda Lonsway I cant even put into words what racing for recovery has helped me improve my life!!!!! It has taught me so much and from that my life has done a complete 180! ❤️#idonteverhavetouseagain

Mary Rimboch McCormick Racing for Recovery is helping my grandson and wife live a positive life without drugs-Your weekly meetings are great-I encourage anyone who has a drug,alcohol,depression or a family who just needs support to make these meetings a must in your life. You will leave with a different out look and definitely a more positive attitude that you can make a change-THANK YOU Racing for Recovery

Rob Crosgrove Gave me tools the tools that I lost in my first recovery gave me hope give me a place to hang out when I had no place give me friends to talk to peers to look up to but most of all gave me recovery

Deanna G Morgan All things are possible🙏❤️💞 Self love, my dad's passing, and putting my boys first! Thank you all! God, self, and my boys is my goal because I want this lifestyle🙏❤️💞 Right on Todd! God bless and have a BEAUTIFUL BLESS day🙏❤️💞😊🌸

Jessica Whitley really I don't even know where to begin with this. I could go on for hours but I will try to express it at the core. Racing helped me realize my happiness isn't forever in the sky. Not only that but happy is so easily attainable through such basic concepts of living. Action, connections, and self worth is all I need to be happy. It demonstrates that from day one of sobriety my dream life is possible. The inspiration I receive from the program creates a consistent drive to keep pursuing whole wellness. It's helped me realize I can be an active, mindful and healthy participante my own life and the actions which accompany that feed the roots of my wellness. I am actually fully alive sometimes even laughing til my face hurts

Deborah Berry Parker Racing has saved my daughters life enough said!!!!!

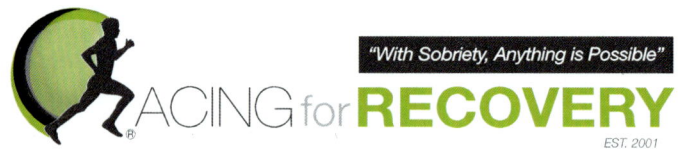